Do-It-Yourself
Allergy Analysis Handbook

Do-It-Yourself Allergy Analysis Handbook

Louise Henderson, Ph.D. and
Kate Ludeman, Ph.D.
with Henry S. Basayne

Keats Publishing, Inc. New Canaan, Connecticut

DO-IT-YOURSELF ALLERGY ANALYSIS HANDBOOK

Copyright © 1979, 1992 by Louise Henderson and
Kate Ludeman
Introduction copyright © 1992 by Doris J. Rapp, M.D.

Library of Congress Cataloging-in-Publication Data

Henderson, Louise.
    Do-it-yourself allergy analysis handbook / Louise
Henderson and Kate Ludeman with Henry S. Basayne.
        p.   cm.
    Ludeman's name appears first on the earlier ed.
    Includes bibliographical references and index.
    ISBN 0-87983-542-7 (pbk.) : $10.95
    1. Allergy—Popular works. I. Ludeman, Kate.
II. Basayne, Henry S. III. Title.
RC584.H43   1991
616.97—dc20   91-16375
                                               CIP

Printed in the United States of America

Keats Publishing, Inc.
27 Pine Street (Box 876), New Canaan, Connecticut 06840

Contents

Introduction

In today's busy, but unfortunately progressively polluted world, many individuals are seeking ways to find more answers which might possibly provide an improved level of health for themselves and their families. Few individuals could pick up this book without recognizing a valuable clue or wanting to try at least a few of the many potentially helpful suggestions.

Probably the only good thing about an allergy is that it is often possible to help yourself by using just a bit of common sense. The key is to learn to think about cause and effect relationships. Always ask about what was eaten, touched or smelled in the hour before your child's or your own illness flared, or before any unusual emotional or activity outburst began.

With the type of basic background information about chemicals and foods mentioned in this book, it is certainly possible to recognize if your problem might be an unrecognized allergy. Allergies can be much more than hay fever, eczema and asthma. The early portion of this book discusses the many faces and facets of allergy and why a single individual's symptoms can change under special circumstances or over time.

One of today's most pressing challenges is to recognize allergies as early as possible in each individual's life. An immense amount of illness and heartache, often starting in infancy and then snowballing right through adulthood, could be prevented if this were done. Of course, you are not physicians and medical expertise should always be sought first if you or your family are not well. Drugs, at times, are essential and they can permanently relieve illness, such as when antibiotic treatment is given for pneumonia. Their continued need, however, indicates that either the cause has not, or cannot, be found.

If the medical professional cannot tell you why you or your child are always ill, there is no rule that says you can't try to figure it out on your own. To quote only one example, recent well-conducted studies indicate that foods can cause epilepsy in some children who also have other medical complaints such as those noted in youngsters who have typical or unusual forms of allergy.[1] In a few years, they may find that a piece of the epilepsy pie can also be caused by dust, pollen, molds and chemicals. Similar studies indicate that arthritis and migraine headaches can be caused by foods in some individuals.[2,3,4] The human body still contains many answers which have at present managed to elude medical detection and understanding.

Once you suspect that an allergy or sensitivity to something might be the cause of your problem, then it is sometimes remarkably easy to determine why you are ill. This small, surprisingly compact book is a gem, brim full of sensible, potentially helpful information for those who choose to try to find and then eliminate the cause of their disease.

This book contains brief, simple descriptions of a number of easily understood concepts related to the scope and possible

1. Egger, J., Soothill, J. 1989. Oligoantigenic diet treatment of children with epilepsy and migraine. *The Journal of Pediatrics* 114(1):51–58.

2. Marshall, R., et al. 1984. Food challenge effects of fasted rheumatoid arthritis patients: A multicenter study. *Clinical Ecology* 2:181–190.

3. Darlington, L., Mansfield, J. 1983. Food allergy and rheumatoid disease. *Annals of the Rheumatic Diseases* 42:218.

4. Egger, J., et al. 1983. Is migraine food allergy? A double-blind controlled trial of oligoantigenic diet treatment. *Lancet* 11:865–869.

causes of the many common, as well as the less frequently recognized forms of allergy. It contains a list of the common symptoms which can influence how some individuals with allergies feel, act, behave and learn. It contains tips about how to prevent or avoid the possible development of future sensitivities. Dietary advice and even recipes are provided. In the section entitled Charts and Lists, there are many bits and pieces of practical information which can be tried on a daily basis to help yourself or your family.

"Learn to live with it" should be the answer only if someone has diligently looked for the cause of an illness. No one really knows you as well as you do, and rarely would anyone spend the time to figure out the answers the way that you would. We must all assume the responsibility of trying to keep ourselves and family well, now and in the future. This book can not only enhance your feeling of well-being but it may well prove to be cost, as well as health, effective. Who could ask for more?

Bless you and may your health improve.

Sincerely,
Doris J. Rapp, M.D.
Buffalo, New York
1992

Do-It-Yourself
Allergy Analysis Handbook

⤎ CHAPTER ONE ⤏

To Begin With . . .

::

YOU ARE WHAT YOU EAT . . . BUT YOU ARE ALSO much *more* than what you eat. The way you live either contributes to your well-being or undermines your health. Nearly all individuals react negatively to some substance—at least for some part of their lives. This sensitivity is commonly called *allergy*.

Allergy is an expression of the body's defenses against substances it does not tolerate well. In years to come, it is likely that the concept of *sensitivity* will replace the word *allergy*. But we will use the word *allergy* here because it is the traditional way to refer to the process of sensitivity reaction.

As individuals, we are perhaps *most* individual in the kinds of things we react to and the ways in which we react. Some people are slightly depressed on days when the sky is overcast; others are indifferent to the weather but respond strongly to particular colors. Are such reactions just in your imagination? We think not. Take the case of someone who tends to cough in movie theaters. The cough could be dismissed as habit or as a psychological quirk. It is likely however, that the dust in theater seats, the smell of popcorn, or the insecticides used in that theater will cause breathing difficulties for someone allergic to dust, corn or insecticide. *It's not your imagination!*

Although the subject of allergy is complex—and although

1

science does not yet fully understand all of your body's allergic responses—we believe that a lot of the mystery can be dispelled. In fact there is a lot you can do to identify and minimize your own sensitivities.

The idea that individuals must take responsibility for their own health is gaining widespread support. More and more, people are seeing their physicians as partners in the process of getting and staying well. The notion that illness seems to come from "out there" and must, therefore, be cured from "out there" is losing hold. We are finding that we can improve our own health with proper rest, exercise, recreation and a reasonable diet, as well as by ancient and innovative approaches from meditation to jogging.

Traditional medicine is essential to the high levels of health care to which we aspire, but it becomes ten times as effective when the patient is well-informed and takes an active part in the process of getting and staying well.

In this book we will describe simple processes by which you can, at home, discover your own allergies and control them. We cannot emphasize strongly enough, however, the value and necessity of guidance by a qualified health care professional. Allergies can be serious. The knowledge, skill and technical know-how of a professional is indispensable. Use it in testing for allergy-producing foods.

Finding the right doctor or other appropriate professional to assist you may not be easy. Some of the theories and methods we describe are still controversial; not all good people in the field agree. Frank discussions with your doctor will reveal objections, levels of understanding, and sympathy or antagonism to your approach. If you want to gain some control over your own health, it's worth the search until you find a professional who understands what you are trying to do and is willing to assist you in doing it.

We want you to learn about allergies and what you can do

about them. We have therefore written this book in a straightforward, non-technical style, even though it touches on complicated theories. Once you've become better-informed we hope that you will be motivated to take charge of your own health by exploring some of the procedures we suggest. This will call for more than a mere change in diet: it will demand real changes in the way you live. Along with increased awareness of your total environment, we hope you will enjoy that high level of well-being, the zest for life, the optimism, energy and joy that are the true measures of good health.

CHAPTER TWO

Do You Have Allergies?

::

YOUR BODY WANTS TO STAY WELL. AN UNBE-lievably sophisticated combination of chemical and electrical systems helps you to grow and maintain your good health. It also warns you when anything threatens your well-being. The pace of modern life, however, has decreased your sensitivity to these warning signals.

If you think of your mind and body as totally separate, you may frequently dismiss mild physical warnings as if they were just mental quirks. For example, if you have a hard time getting up in the morning, do you respond by thinking ''that's just the way I am''? Fatigue, especially chronic fatigue, is an early warning signal that all is not well. Your body may not be getting something it needs, or it may be gearing up to resist an oncoming illness. When you experience chronic fatigue, you exist in that common, low-level state of health in which you are not really *ill*, but not really well, either.

Great numbers of other symptoms, some quite vague, frequently are signals that you are sensitive to food, pollen or chemicals. For instance, are you especially sensitive to odors? Do you react strongly to changes in weather? Do you frequently feel cold when others around you are comfortable?

Do you have strong aversions, or uncontrollable cravings, for certain foods? Do you bruise easily?

You can help your body regain or maintain good health by learning to recognize these signals, relating them to possible environmental causes and avoiding those things that make you react.

Like a small child who wants attention, your body sends increasingly stronger signals if the early ones are ignored. If you don't respond to a mild warning, such as a skin rash or hives, the signals become more urgent. You may begin to suffer from diarrhea or headache. If you *still* fail to respond, physical fire bells go off and you may develop asthma or even more drastic symptoms.

The process of increasing physical warnings is long and slow. Although you may sustain some low-grade discomfort, weeks, months or even years may pass before the next symptom level appears.

If you add some kind of acute stress to a mild malaise, it can trigger a rapid escalation of symptoms. Stress may come from a violent, external and sudden change; but it can also result from subtle changes in lifestyle. For example, after a job change (and/or a change in working conditions) you will be subject not only to new emotional stresses, but also possibly to a new chemical environment, one to which your body may react negatively. Pregnancy alters hormone balances, which can result in increased sensitivity to food and chemicals. Mental or emotional discomfort to which you are exposed over a period of time—such as marital discord or financial problems— can provide the stress that leads to a more severe degree of physical reaction.

When you react in some new way to a commonly occurring substance or situation, you are experiencing an *allergic reaction*. Clearly, there is great value in learning to recognize and respond to the early, minor levels of warning from your body. When you understand the cause of your sensitivity, you can avoid it and prevent a series of increasingly severe responses by your body.

CHAPTER THREE

What is Allergy?

::

ALLERGY IS YOUR BODY'S NATURAL DEFENSE against any threat by a foreign substance. Like a fortress under seige, the attack upon your body stimulates a series of defensive measures.

Your body has two basic defense systems. The first, the *thymico-lymphatic system*, uses two fundamental strategies: the *immune* and the *inflammatory* responses. The second, the *endocrine system,* engages key regulatory glands in your body: your thyroid and adrenals. Your body's immune sequence works something like this:

The foreign invader (an *antigen*) is detected by the scouts of your immune army (*T-cells*). They report the enemy action, and the generals send battle instructions to the platoon leaders (*B-cells*). The platoon leaders produce infantry (*antibodies*, sometimes called *immunoglobulins*). These antibodies do the actual fighting for your immune army. If the battle is not going well—if they seem to be losing and need some help—a call may go out for the atomic bomb of your immune system (the *complement*). As with nuclear weapons, your body's immune system operates on a fail-safe system in which certain events must occur in a particular order before the big blast goes off. Also, as with a nuclear weapon, the complement is not a very discriminating instrument. It works by blasting a hole in the

7

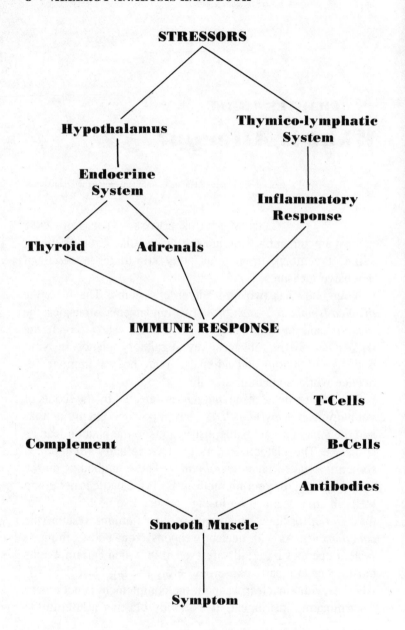

cell so that the destructive enzymes will leak out, clearing the antigen or invader. But it can also damage healthy cells in the process.

When any substance (*antigen*) that is not an inherent part of your body tries to enter it, the body tries to protect itself by producing antibodies. This sequence of natural physical defenses makes up the immune system; allergy is thus a response of the immune system.

The inflammatory response is another strategy this system uses to resist foreign invaders. When you suffer an insect bite or a splinter under the skin, the protective response involves inflammation, redness and swelling. When resistance has developed to a significant extent however, the inflammation can damage the body it is trying to protect. To control this, the body activates its own anti-inflammatory response.

Bear in mind that the inflammatory and immune responses are reactions to invaders of that thymico-lymphatic line of defense. The *endocrine* line of defense (which can also engage the immune response) is the other basic way the body responds to the stress of an allergen.

Stress is a necessary and valuable part of your life, but it can also be potentially destructive. Although its evolutionary purpose is to protect you from danger and ensure your survival, repeated or sustained stress can be devastating.

Suppose you are a prehistoric cave person. A sabre-toothed tiger sees you and prepares to dine. You see *it*, and the stress of your plight puts a rapid, dramatic and life-saving sequence of events into motion inside your body. The brain tells the adrenal glands to secrete a particular hormone (a glucocortocoid). This causes the protein-building blocks (the amino acids) to be redistributed in the body. Muscle tone increases, blood pressure and respiration levels increase, body-repair mechanisms are put on red alert and all the defense systems of the body are mobilized. You are now physically ready either to combat the danger or to flee from it. This, the "fight or flight" response, is a marvelously useful mechanism when facing a sabre-toothed tiger or other life-threatening situation. But if the cause of stress is less clear-cut—if it comes from something as unpleasant as constant disapproving looks from your boss—the continued production of these hormones can have a damaging effect on you. In fact, chronic stress can cause high blood pressure, ulcers or even actual degeneration of lymphatic tissue.

This theory of chronic stress, its benefits and its dangers was developed by Dr. Hans Selye. He called it the "general adaptation syndrome." According to Selye, stage one is the alarm reaction; stage two, the mobilizing of resistance; and stage three—if the stress-producing stimulus is not soon removed—the stage of exhaustion, in which the body's own repair system can begin to damage itself.

The "fight or flight" reaction is an example of the endocrine defense in action. A key element in this defense may be the production of hormones by the pituitary and adrenal glands. The defense may go awry, however, and under- or over-production results. This kind of reaction may involve the body's *sympathetic nervous system*, which controls involuntary muscle activity and leads to the "fight or flight" response, or *para-sympathetic nervous system*, which leads to exhaustion and breakdown (stage three of Selye's general adaptation syndrome).

Stress load is well expressed in the familiar story of the camel and the last straw. Your body can bear the weight of just so much before it shows symptoms of discomfort and pain. If the weight keeps growing, despite these complaints, the body finally crumples under the burden. You interact with your environment constantly—the food you eat, the air you breathe, the water you drink (and the chemicals in each of them)—and each adds weight to the cargo your body is struggling to manage. Your household environment, job, clothing, relationships—all contribute to the demands upon you. Other factors, like pollen, dust, molds and chemicals—even barometric pressure, outside temperature and pollution levels—add to the stress on your body and may finally cause allergic reactions. You are usually well equipped to handle these demands without becoming sick. But if the stress load becomes too great, your body protests; the result can be any kind of physical or psychological symptom.

How can an antigen or stress attack in one part of the body affect other body systems? When an allergic reaction occurs, the affected cells give off hydrogen ions, causing the extracellular fluid to become more acidic. Normally, this fluid is in a delicate balance of acidity and alkalinity. (Normal acid level is designated as pH 7.36.) In response to an antigen, this now highly acidic fluid may be triggered by one of the factors of the immune system, irritating other cells with which it comes in contact.

The increase and accumulation of such fluid in a particular part of the body is called *edema*. The swelling of edema can cause your normally well-fitting ring to feel tight and uncomfortable, or your eyes to become puffy, or your ankles and feet to swell. Even the brain can pick up excess, irritating fluid from this reaction. If many cells react to an antigen in this fashion, entire organs and body systems may respond with pain.

The smooth muscle system may also cause an allergic response throughout the body. Smooth muscle groups in nearly every part of the body work in close relationship to the intricate and extensive network of blood vessels. There are four major groups of smooth muscles. An antigen attack on the *respiratory system* group can result in sinusitis, bronchitis, asthma or—in severe cases—respiratory failure. An unwelcome invader in the *gastrointestinal system* may result in inflammation of the esophagus, the stomach or intestines. You may consequently suffer from spasms, colitis, diarrhea or constipation as an allergic response. If the immune system is activated in the *genitourinary system*, you may experience is as cystitis, vaginitis, chronic inflammation of the uterus, ovaries or urethra. Headaches of all kinds, phlebitis, bruising or even cardiac involvement or failure can be caused by an allergic immune system reaction in the *vascular system*, the blood circulation network.

You can see why it is sometimes very difficult to identify the symptoms of an allergic response. Symptoms vary within each of the body's systems, and more than one system may become involved at the same time. Multiple-system response is often caused by the same sensitivity occurring over and over—the physical reaction to a repeated stress stimulus.

Mild reactions, such as sinus fullness, sneezing or watery eyes that occur in hay fever antigen response may be neutralized by the use of antihistamines or shots to combat the invader. Unfortunately, most sensitivity reactions are not quite so clear cut.

Although initial symptoms may be very mild and go unnoticed, symptoms will become progressively worse if exposure to the offending agent continues. This intensification of symptoms is known as a cascade or "crescendo" effect.

We have said that when your body is assaulted repeatedly by the same stress factors or antigens, and the same reaction occurs over and over, a disease process is established. If the disease is diagnosed, a medication may be prescribed. But how else could you manage such a disease? What if you were able to identify the cause of a particular, unwelcome body response, and learn to avoid it? By preventing the repetition of symptoms, your body might be able to return to its normal state of well-being; the disease might never have a chance to become established.

⌘§ CHAPTER FOUR ❧

What Are the Symptoms of Allergy?

::

PEOPLE RARELY BECOME ILL ALL AT once. Usually there are signs and symptoms snowballing with each year. The signs are supposed to tell us something is wrong. Consider this case history which is exaggerated so that even those not accustomed to the trickery of allergy can see the progression.

When Joe was fifteen, he developed a skin rash and nasal inflammation during the fall of each year. He was treated with antihistamines. At age twenty, while in college, he suffered eyestrain and took aspirin for relief. At twenty-five, Joe developed an ulcer and was placed on a bland diet. At thirty, he noticed numbness and tingling sensations in his hands and head. A doctor diagnosed his condition as hypoglycemic and prescribed a high-protein diet. At age thirty-three, Joe took a job as an accountant in a factory that made batteries. There he was constantly exposed to chemical fumes. After six months he began to suffer blackouts and chest pains. The next year, Joe had strong arrhythmic heart palpitations and sharp chest pains. Two heart attacks followed two years later.

The sequence of symptoms of increasing severity—the "crescendo effect"—is very clear. And the hint exists in this dismal recital that poor Joe suffered from a never-diagnosed addiction to certain foods. We'll have more to say about addiction later.

When Joe was fifteen he experienced hay fever symptoms, probably because of various pollens and molds in his environment. The antihistamine prescribed did nothing to eliminate the cause of his problem, and a disease process was established by repeated exposure and response.

His headaches, resulting from skipped meals, suggest that he had begun an addictive eating pattern which was unrecognized. With the milk-heavy bland food diet and the high protein hypoglycemic diet, he had very little variety in his food intake during those periods. The repetition of these foods, and his predisposition to food allergy, intensified the addictive pattern and it became chronic.

Some allergic reactions are clear cut—you may break out in hives whenever you eat strawberries. But other allergic reactions are more insidious; these typically mimic the patterns of addiction. You may be surprised at the relationship of allergy to addiction, but a person can develop an addiction to the very substance to which he or she is sensitive. When the body is forced to keep on accepting a food or other antigen that it can no longer tolerate, it adapts as best it can. It tries to maintain a state as close to normal as possible in the presence of the offending invader. This forced adaptation can lead to physical addiction, because the body now *requires* the presence of the antigen in order to function at its near-normal level. If the body misses its expected dose of the antigen, it goes into withdrawal, intensifying the symptoms. Re-introducing the addicting substance into the body once again will temporarily relieve the symptoms and make the addict feel better—for a short while. As a result, as an addict (whether the addiction is to tobacco, hard drugs or particular food), you may actually crave the very substance that is responsible for your chronic symptoms. You may never suspect the cause and effect relationship between that substance and your illness.

This addictive process in allergy is similar to alcohol and other drug addictions. The initial response is stimulation, followed by the body's need for greater and greater quantities of the stimulant in order to achieve the same effect. Ultimately, as an addict, you reach a point where you are no longer stimulated by your ''fix.'' In this state, a person feels awful in contact with the addictive substance, but worse without it.

You probably think of most addictive substances as poisons—as indeed they are. The build up of allergens in the body is also very much like being poisoned. As the toxic level rises, the body systems break down further. A wide variety of physical or psychological symptoms may result. Do your muscles feel stiff, tense or aching? Have you considered that allergy may be the cause? What about swelling or redness in your joints? You know about sneezing, eye-watering and nasal stuffiness as a response to hay fever and other pollen-caused allergies, but did you realize that these may also result from certain foods you eat? A rapid heartbeat or throbbing pulse or a sharp chest pain may be caused by an allergen as can urinary or genital discomfort, or the urge to urinate without the need.

Common allergic responses include stomach distress, burping and, in more severe reactions, nausea or acute cramping. If you always (or never) seem to be hungry, consider the possibility of allergic reaction. Excessive sweating, itching skin or sallow complexion may also come from allergens. Sore and swollen throats and difficulty in swallowing can be added to the list, as can word-reversal, not quite being able to find the words you want or other speech coordination problems.

Sharp, throbbing or dull headaches and migraines may be a body warning of allergic reaction. And if you are super-sensitive to odors—or absolutely insensitive to them—allergy may be suspected. Ears that ache or ears that itch are frequently the result of sensitivity to allergens, and a ringing in the ears can be similarly caused.

It is also appropriate to suspect allergy as the root cause of hypersensitivity to light, blurred vision, itchy or watery eyes. And people rarely connect deep, dark circles under the eyes with allergic response, but it is a very common symptom.

Sleep disturbances, whether insomnia, nightmares, excessive drowsiness or common, constant fatigue, may well be allergic reactions. Feelings of lightheadedness, fainting, poor attention span, mental confusion and agitation also indicate allergy.

When, without apparent cause, someone you know seems severely depressed, despairing or sad, or particularly irritable, tense or sharp with others, it is worth considering that these behaviors may result from allergies.

Obviously, all these symptoms may have other causes. But you should be aware that allergy is also a possible source of these reactions, and only recently have some of these connections been recognized. For instance, research has now shown that hyperactivity in some children can be directly related to the way they react to the colorings and preservatives in their food. Removal of these allergens from their diets results in nearly immediate calming.

The stereotypes of allergy symptoms are asthma, hay fever and rashes, but many changes in mood and behavior are also responses of the immune system. These psychological reactions are related to what happens in the body. The brain is the source of psychological behavior, but it is also a physical organ that responds with allergy to unwelcome stimuli, as do the other organs of the body. You are both body *and* mind, and each affects the other. Where allergy is concerned, even psychological response is not your imagination; it may be physical in origin.

Imagine a line that stretches from severe depression on one end to manic hyperactivity on the other. In the middle is the kind of healthy, zestful, fully alive feeling to which we all aspire. Our behavior on this midline is at an even keel.

Moving one step toward the depression end of the scale there are some local, physical manifestations of allergy: running or stuffy nose, eczema or hives, colitis and asthma. Moving another step toward depression, the system displays physical and psychological responses such as tiredness, mild depression, edema, backache or muscle and joint inflammation. The next level of depression can result in noticeably disturbed behavior: confusion, indecisiveness, moodiness, apathy. In a more advanced degree a person will show impairment of comprehension and attention and may suffer mental lapses and blackouts. At the far end, a severe depression may be expressed as lethargy, disorientation, delusions, amnesia and paranoia. At worst, the severely depressed person will become comatose.

Starting again from the happy midpoint of our mood and physical scale, move one level toward the ''up'' end. A person in this stimulated state will be relatively symptom free and appear active, alert, lively and responsive. Such a person will frequently display energy, initiative and wit, and will tend to be considerate of others. Our society puts a high value on this level of behavior.

But it is just another step from this desirable state to hyperactivity and irritability. Those who function at this level of stimulation may show physical responses such as acute hunger or thirst, flushing, sweating and chilling, insomnia or obesity. In terms of behavior, we see such a person as hopped up, jittery, tense, talkative, supersensitive and self-centered.

The next level toward hyperactivity can be recognized by

++++ MANIC WITH OR WITHOUT CONVULSIONS	Distraught, excited, agitated, enraged and panicky. Circuitous or one-track thoughts, muscle twitching and jerking of extremities, convulsive seizures and altered consciousness may develop.	**Maladapted Advanced Stimulatory Responses**
+++ HYPOMANIC, TOXIC, ANXIOUS AND EGOCENTRIC	Aggressive, loquacious, clumsy (ataxic), anxious, fearful and apprehensive; alternating chills and flushing, ravenous hunger, excessive thirst. Giggling or pathological laughter may occur.	
++ HYPERACTIVE, IRRITABLE, HUNGRY AND THIRSTY	Tense, jittery, hopped up, talkative, argumentative, sensitive, overly responsive, self-centered, hungry and thirsty; flushing, sweating and chilling may occur as well as insomnia, alcoholism and obesity.	**Adapted Responses**
+ STIMULATED BUT RELATIVELY SYMPTOM FREE	Active, alert, lively, responsive and enthusiastic with unimpaired ambition, energy, initiative and wit. Considerate of the views and actions of others. This usually comes to be regarded as "normal" behavior.	
0 BEHAVIOR ON AN EVEN KEEL AS IN HOMEOSTASIS	Children expect this from their parents and teachers. Parents expect this from their children. We all expect this from our associates.	

Maladapted Localized Responses	Maladapted Systemic Responses	Maladapted Cerebral and Behavioral Responses	
—LOCALIZED ALLERGIC MANIFESTATIONS	— —SYSTEMIC ALLERGIC MANIFESTATIONS	– – –BRAIN-FAG, MILD DEPRESSION AND DISTURBED THINKING	– – – –SEVERE DEPRESSION WITH OR WITHOUT ALTERED CONSCIOUSNESS
Running or stuffy nose, clearing throat, coughing, wheezing (asthma), itching (eczema and hives), gas, diarrhea, constipation (colitis), urgency and frequency of urination and various eye and ear syndromes.	Tired, dopey, somnolent, mildly depressed, edematous with painful syndromes (headache, neckache, backache, neuralgia, myalgia, myositis, arthralgia, arthritis, chest pain) and cardiovascular effects.*	Confused, indecisive, moody, sad, sullen, withdrawn or apathetic. Emotional instability and impaired attention, concentration, comprehension and thought processes (aphasia, mental lapse and blackouts).	Nonresponsive, lethargic, stuporous, disoriented, melancholic, incontinent, regressive thinking, paranoid orientation, delusions, hallucinations, sometimes amnesia and coma.

anxious behavior, aggressiveness, fearfulness and apprehension. Such persons may be hypertalkative and clumsy, and experience ravenous hunger and excessive thirst.

The most extreme level of manic hyperactivity may occur with or without convulsions. Muscle twitching, jerking of the extremities, persistent one-track thoughts and circuitous thinking patterns—are all typical of someone in this state. Such persons are agitated, easily excited or enraged, or distraught, and they may experience altered states of consciousness.

CHAPTER FIVE

What Are the Sources of Allergy?

::

THE DIFFERENCES AMONG PEOPLE ARE GREATER than their similarities. Although everyone may be allergic to some substances, they certainly are not all susceptible to the same things or to the same degree. People have different genetic heritages and different metabolic rates.

Your immune system is unique. The things that trigger its response are not necessarily those that will trigger the immune system in the person next to you. Some people are highly allergic to poison oak or poison ivy; others you know can tramp happily through a field of poison ivy with nary an itch or rash.

Potential allergens are everywhere around you—in the foods you eat, the pollens carried in the air you breathe, in the multitude of chemicals that permeate your environment. If your body has to keep defending itself against one particular allergen, you are likely to become increasingly sensitive to other allergens. Conversely, if you are able to bring your major allergic responses under control, you will probably enjoy increased resistance to the remaining allergens.

For example, if you can avoid those foods and chemicals that make you respond with severe symptoms, you may, at the same time, reduce your sensitivity to pollens. Pollens don't lend themselves easily to avoidance, which is the fundamental treatment method proposed in this handbook. Therefore, the book will not deal with pollen allergies. But remember, as your general health improves and your resistance increases, you are less likely to suffer allergic effects from *any* source.

Chemical Allergy

Chemicals play an essential role in today's society. The automobile you drive, the storage of your food, the manufacture of your clothing all rely on the chemicals and compounds that are now universal on and around the planet Earth. Hundreds of thousands of chemicals abound in our modern world, and they are being added to at the rate of about two thousand new compounds and synthetics each year. But these chemicals, helpful as they are, constitute a massive assault on your body.

The human body has evolved slowly over millions of years. The gradual process of human adaptation to the environment, enabling humans to survive and thrive, cannot keep pace with the *rate* of change in the atmosphere caused by our accelerating use of synthetic chemicals. Perhaps in time the species may adapt and learn to accommodate these new pollutants, but *you* don't have thousands, or even hundreds, of years to get used to them. So you must become aware that, despite their usefulness, chemicals may represent a major source of your allergic reaction.

Chemicals are used in crop production, in the manufacture of fabrics and in food preservation. Among the many other uses for chemicals are some which you can, and probably should, avoid. Manufacturers are increasingly concerned about the effects of their chemically-loaded products, and some are taking steps to reduce the hazards. But certain synthetic chemicals, for instance, have now been shown capable of producing cancer in humans. It is up to you to be alert to those chemical sources that have allergic or toxic effects on your body.

The highest chemical levels that you encounter are in your own home. Synthetic carpets and fabrics, foam furniture, cleaning aids, air fresheners—these and hundreds of other chemically-based products are a constant element in the biosphere. One study of air pollution shows that the concentration of chemical contaminants is 400 times greater in the home than in the outside air.

Formaldehyde is the most common chemical in the average household. It is a highly active compound that exists in nature as a gas. By itself it has little odor, but it can cause a burning sensation in the eyes and mucous membranes. It is produced in large amounts as a by-product of internal combustion engines and is probably responsible for the burning sensation associated with high smog levels.

Formaldehyde is used as an intermediate in the synthesis of alcohols, acids and other chemicals. It is also used as a tanning agent, in the manufacture of concrete and plaster, as an antiperspirant, and as an antiseptic in toothpaste, mouthwash and germicidal and detergent soaps. You will also find formaldehyde in hairsetting preparations and shampoos. Since it destroys bacteria, fungus, molds and yeast, it is frequently used as a disinfectant in hospitals, in the manufacture of antibiotics and in the fermentation industries.

Formaldehyde is a principal component of embalming fluid and is used to preserve waxes, polishes, adhesives, fats and oils. It is also found in explosives, fireproofing compounds, compositions applied to fabrics, in the synthesis of dyes, and in solutions for killing insects and rodents. It improves the wet strength of paper products and is found in photographic developing solutions, nail polish, wallboard and resins. It makes both natural and synthetic fibers crease resistant, crushproof, dyefast, flame- and water-resistant, shrinkproof, mothproof and more elastic. The aldehydes constitute a major portion of the pollutants in the air that now covers the earth. Formaldehyde represents about half of the aldehydes in such air. High levels are produced by the gasoline engine, coal, fuel oil and natural gas combustion, petroleum refining and incineration.

The second most frequently encountered chemical is *chlorine*. In its pure form, chlorine gas is a deadly poison. It binds readily with other chemicals in compounds. It is frequently used for water purification, sterilization, bleaching and as an anesthetic. It is found in textiles and paper pulp, cleaning fluid, disinfectants and many drugs. It is used in the refining of both oil and sugar.

Phenol is the third most common chemical group. In its pure form, it is also called carbolic acid or hydroxybenzine and chemically resembles the alcohol group of chemicals.

Phenol's antiseptic properties were used by Joseph Lister in the treatment of wounds as early as 1845. The simple phenols are liquids with extremely high boiling points. Unlike formaldehyde and natural gas, which have little or no odor, the phenols have an easily-detected characteristic odor. The phenols are found in nature as the toxic agents in poison ivy and poison oak, and in spring water near coal and oil deposits.

One form, called "cresol" (methylphenol), is an extremely effective antiseptic and disinfectant; this form accounts for our highest immediate levels of exposure, particularly from products like Lysol and Pinesol. Phenol is found in epoxy resins, aspirin and other drugs and in herbicides and pesticides. It is used in the manufacture of nylon, explosives, detergents, polyurethane, perfume and gasoline. It is also a preservative found in medications, including allergy shots.

The *alcohols* are the fourth most common source of chemical antigens in our environment. Throughout history they have been used as antiseptics and solvents and for human consumption. Ethyl alcohol is used as a solvent in the manufacture of toilet and drug preparations, and in the making of rubber and ether. Amyl alcohol is frequently used as a solvent. Isopropyl alcohol is found in antifreeze, rubbing alcohol and solvents. Glycerol is used for sweetening and preserving foods, in the manufacture of cosmetics, perfumes, inks, glue and cement, and in skin emollients. Menthol is used in liquors, confections, perfumes and cold remedies. Alcohol is also used as a source of light and heat, as a motor fuel, a disinfectant and a sedative.

Perfumes are another common source of chemical antigens. They are now commonly found in facial tissue, toilet paper, lipsticks and other cosmetics, soap, body deodorants, air fresheners and candles.

Expensive perfumes are usually derived from rare flower oils, but the perfumes in soap and the less expensive types are made from synthetic materials. Most are blends of flower oil, animal substances, synthetics, alcohol and water.

Plant oil is extracted by steam distillation. Animal substances are obtained by slow evaporation: castor from the beaver, musk from the male musk deer, ambergris from the sperm whale. Other materials come from coal tar and petrochemicals. Alcohol is added to these elements and heated; then the mixture is diluted with water.

The three basic types of perfume are extracts (also called essences), colognes and toilet water. Essences contain up to 20 percent perfume, dissolved in alcohol. Colognes may contain 3 to 5 percent perfume oil and 80 to 90 percent alcohol, with water making up the balance. Toilet water is about 2 percent perfume and 60 to 80 percent alcohol; the rest is water.

Insecticides represent another frequent source of allergy-producing chemicals. The high level of food production and the extraordinary American crop yield per acre depend on the use of insecticides. But the poisons used to deter insects from eating your food before it gets off the farm are toxic not only to food pests but to animals and humans as well. Some insecticides have had such a devastating effect on the environment and the food-chain that they have been banned by the government; DDT is a prime example.

Insecticides are sprayed on plants before the fruit, grain or vegetables sprout or bud. The chemicals are therefore incorporated into the plant cells as the plant grows. Since the insecticide is in the plant cell system, washing it off the surface does little good. When a susceptible individual eats the plant, he eats the insecticide as well.

Household pesticides are frequently put in a petroleum base to give the poisons more durability in controlling insects and rodents. The result is that a bug may be exposed to such an insecticide for a longer period of time, but so is the human being who is trying to get rid of the bug. A large number of products you use may have residual insecticides or fungicides: tobacco, rubber products (including rubber bands), packing boxes, wool products and grocery store produce. If you are allergic to pesticides, you should avoid areas such as orchards, farms, riding stables, storerooms, theaters and garden shops.

Food Allergy

Conventional wisdom has it that ''one man's meat is another man's poison.'' As you may have discovered, this can be painfully and literally true. Most animals have some level of instinct that protects them from ingesting foods that are bad for them. Humans, by and large, have overridden this protective mechanism and, with the encouragement of bright and clever packaging, advertising slogans and the perfection of sales persuasion techniques, tend to eat a lot of things that are not nutritious, and in some cases are downright harmful.

How is it that even wholesome and nutritious foods can act like poisons for some people? How can fresh fish, rich in protein and a staple of life in many cultures, cause acute allergic shock in some hypersensitive individuals? Why is it that milk fresh from the dairy can turn a charming, rosy infant into a howling demon? How can a single nut, or even the smell of a nut, make a grown man wheeze and gasp for breath? It's easy to understand that food gone bad can act like a veritable poison; that spoiled foods can harbor devastating and sometimes fatal bacteria (such as that which causes botulism); that certain foods, like peppers, garlic or onions, might be difficult for some people to digest. But it is very difficult to realize that good, fresh food can cause some reactive people deep distress, with a host of both physical and psychological symptoms.

Science is a long way from explaining everything about allergy, but allergy is generally thought to work in two main ways: by direct contact of food allergens with antibodies in the digestive system, resulting in swift reactions, or by the absorption of allergens into the blood stream from the digestive tract, resulting in skin, blood, smooth muscle, glandular and mucous membrane reactions.

Nearly everyone is sensitive to some substance at some time in their lives; nearly everyone has experienced at least a mild allergic response—passing indigestion, stuffy nose, brief irritability or depression. And nearly any food can cause allergy. The most common allergenic foods are corn, wheat, milk, beef, eggs, potatoes and sugar. Since allergy can act like addiction, it's no coincidence that these are the foods most often eaten by Americans, regularly or even daily. Our bodies, in fact, are overloaded with these foods and food by-products. Although each of these foods is a valuable source of important nutrients, the nutritional benefit is more than cancelled out if the food causes severe allergic reaction.

In recent years, the laws that require the listing of ingredients on food product labels have served thoughtful people; you not only learn what it is you are eating, you can use that information to avoid products that contain foods to which you are allergic. You owe it to yourself to develop the habit of reading labels before you buy any labelled product. There are some foods, like freshly-baked cakes, that aren't labelled, of course. When you discover that you are reactive to a particular food, it is worth your while to learn where it may be hiding.

Take pastries and cakes, for example. Suppose you know that you are allergic to *yeast*. It's reasonable to expect that yeast will usually be found in bread, cake, crackers, hot dog buns and pretzels. But did you suspect that yeast was also used in the manufacture of many vitamins (especially the B-complex), whiskey, soy sauce, sour cream, ginger ale, cheese and beer?

If you are hypersensitive to *corn* (maize), you need to know that corn products may be found in adhesives (such as gummed envelopes and stamps), aspirin, baking powder, breath sprays, many carbonated beverages and processed cereals. And corn is frequently an ingredient in chewing gum, instant coffee, cream puffs and paper cups. Worse, you can be exposed to corn by inhaling fumes from cooking corn, ironing starched clothes and applying body powders. Glucose and dextrose sweeteners and many medications may also contain corn or corn derivatives, as do processed fried foods, gelatin desserts, graham crackers, hot dogs and hair sprays. Most lollipops are made from corn syrup; MSG and plastic food wrappers are corn carriers; and so are pickles and processed rice. Seasoning salt, sausage, spaghetti, toothpaste and some canned, creamed and frozen vegetables—all are sources of allergy for those sensitive to corn.

Milk can often be an allergen. Of course, those who react to milk will avoid malted milk, condensed milk, evaporated milk and dried milk, but will you think to avoid the things that are commonly made with milk—waffles, doughnuts, biscuit mixes and mashed potatoes? How about au gratin foods, bologna, butter and cheese? Most candy has milk products, as do processed salad dressings, sherbets and soda crackers.

Even *wheat*, the staff of life, can raise havoc with your system if you are allergic to it. Did you know that it may show up in beer, bourbon or scotch? It's also frequently found in breads, including corn bread, gluten, pumpernickel, rye and soy—not just wheat breads. Cereals and flours obviously contain wheat, but not so obvious is the fact that buckwheat, a member of the rhubarb family and not a wheat, is often mixed with wheat when it is packaged. Other sources of wheat exposure are bouillon cubes, liverwurst, ice cream thickeners and malted milks and candies.

Alcoholic beverages may also be a source of grain exposure, but not always the ones you think. Bourbon usually contains corn, malt and rye, and may contain wheat, oats and/or rice, as well. While imported vodka is made from potatoes, domestic vodka may include corn, rye and wheat. Irish whiskey and beer both frequently contain rice. You'll find an interesting chart about the food constituents of alcoholic beverages in the section called Charts and Lists at the back of this book.

ᴥᔄ CHAPTER SIX ᔅᴥ

What Can You Do about Allergy?

::

WHEN YOU HAVE A PARTICULARLY UNCOMFORT-able symptom, you can often get temporary relief with medication. But how much better it would be if you could identify the cause of the problem!

The diagnosis of allergy is often difficult: you may be responding to more than one allergen, your sensitivity may be to some substance (like an insecticide) that isn't readily apparent in the food you are testing, and/or a number of body systems can be involved in many allergic reactions.

Several methods are commonly used to diagnose or treat allergies. The most frequently used are *cytotoxic blood testing, provocative testing* and the *elimination diet*. Some less traditional methods are *exercise, muscle testing* and *ortho-molecular therapy*. In many cases, the treatment method is closely related to the diagnosis method.

We once again urge you to consult a physician or other qualified health care professional for guidance in identifying or treating an allergic condition. Some allergic reactions can be quite severe; sympathetic and skilled professionals can help you avoid serious trouble and assist you in the event of unanticipated reactions.

The *cytotoxic blood test* is used only to diagnose your body's response to specific foods. A sample of your white cells is mixed with a small amount of the food being tested and added to a culture of blood components. This process reveals whether or not your white cells produce antibodies against that food. Your physician can also judge the level of your response to the food using this method. A disadvantage of this test is that it may be invalid if you also suffer from chemical sensitivity. If you do, this test is not definitive because the extract being tested may contain preservatives and other chemicals. Obviously, the cytotoxic tests can only be performed by a professional.

Provocative testing is of two types. In provocative *skin* testing, a small amount or concentrate of the suspected substance is injected under your skin, usually on your arm. With the antigen introduced directly into the body, antibody and other reactions may be provoked and easily observed.

In a typical reaction, a weal of irritation or inflammation appears on the skin at the site of the injection. By observing the size of the weal your physician is able to estimate the level of your reaction to the solution. Some people don't react distinctly in this fashion, and for them, the *sublingual* method may better reveal the source of their allergies.

In *sublingual testing* (sublingual is Latin for "under the tongue") a few drops of the suspected food or chemical are placed directly under the tongue. Absorption into the blood stream is very rapid, and your doctor watches for reactive symptoms. In provocative testing, especially in the sublingual method, response to the testing solution may cause a set of symptoms to rapidly appear that mimic the symptoms you have in response to that substance—a runny nose or a slight depression.

Variations of the same methods are also used in treatment. You are given neutralizing doses of the allergen, either by injection or under the tongue, until the gradually decreasing dosages neutralize you to the offending substance.

Desensitization injections are also used in the treatment of pollen, mold or other inhaled allergy-producing substances. The "soup" with which you're injected is tailor-made, especially compounded of those materials to which you react, in a dosage appropriate for you. Again, obviously, the provocative testing and treatment methods require the services of your physician.

It may surprise you to consider *exercise* as a therapy for allergy, but you will recall that one of the ways allergies develop throughout your body is through smooth muscle and the lymphatic system. The circulatory network of blood vessels—veins and arteries—carries irritated and irritating cells to the affected organs where the toxins tend to build up. With increased blood flow, fresh oxygenated blood is brought in increasing quantity to these areas, and the debris—the toxins—are carried off. So the area is both nourished and cleansed by the speed-up of blood flow, and the veins and arteries become healthier and more elastic with the increased supply of rich blood.

When you engage in strenuous exercise, your respiration and blood pressure increase; your whole system speeds up. Synaptic transmission—the means your body uses to transmit nerve impulses—is also elevated, so you think and respond more efficiently. Exercise has the additional advantage of generating perspiration, which is another effective system for getting rid of poisons. Regular, strenuous (but not *too* strenuous) exercise improves over-all health and body functions and can be a key, continuing method to help your body rid itself of allergy-caused toxins. Be sure to get professional advice about the best kind of exercise for you.

A simple, self-administered testing procedure is called *kinesiology*, or muscle testing. While this method has not been thoroughly researched and is, therefore, still controversial, it is not hazardous and seems to work for many people. The underlying theory relies on a view of the body as a whole, so that what affects one part may, in turn, affect all. As a consequence, any food or chemical placed in the mouth may cause a reaction in the muscle systems. In this diagnostic method, muscle strength is first established. For example, the thumb and index finger are pressed together; then the amount of resistance it takes to prevent them from being pulled apart is measured. A food such as chocolate or coffee is then taken into the mouth, and the muscle is immediately re-tested. If there is much less resistance, an allergy to that food may be suspected. By gentle manipulation of balancing muscles, and by tracing nerve, circulatory or other body systems (meridians), this theory says that muscle resistance can be increased and balanced, and general good health can be restored.

Another emerging method of allergy treatment is called *orthomolecular* therapy. ''Ortho-'' means straight, right or proper, and this method attempts to raise the general health level through nutrition. Sometimes referred to as megavitamin therapy, it frequently involves high, therapeutic dosages of minerals and enzymes as well as vitamins. Where there has been a long history of chronic illness or stress, even a wholesome diet may not provide all the nutrients needed for the good health and high performance of all the body systems. Orthomolecular therapy seeks to restore biochemical balance. This study of vitamins and their interaction, and the administration of high dosages of appropriate substances, has proven effective for many people in allergy treatment. The nutrients most commonly used in this process are vitamins A, B_1, B_2, B_6, B_{12}, C, D, E, calcium pantothenate and folic acid, and the minerals calcium, magnesium, manganese and zinc.

Many vitamins advertised as pure or organic also contain fillers, binders and other non-vitamin materials, such as cornstarch. You may be sensitive to these substances, called excipients, so you need to know what's actually in each pill. Since some vitamins are stored in the body, and high levels may actually be toxic, consult your physician when planning a vitamin regimen.

Food and chemical testing that you can do yourself (with professional guidance) is a complex subject. By cleansing the system and methodically testing individual foods and chemicals you can identify those which cause your allergic reactions. By eliminating the offending substances from your diet and environment you avoid the allergic reaction and, over a period of time, your body frequently loses its sensitivity to that allergen. It is a method that we want to explain in detail, so it gets the next chapter all to itself.

❄§ CHAPTER SEVEN ৪❄

How Can You Avoid Allergens?

::

YOUR BEST PROTECTION AGAINST ALLERGY IS to avoid the foods or chemicals that cause it; such an avoidance must be total. The *elimination diet* is a testing method that first eliminates all potential allergens from your system: food, chemicals, etc. After the old allergens are cleared from the body by fasting, you expose yourself—one at a time—to suspected foods and chemicals. By carefully monitoring your own body and the symptoms that may develop, you can identify your sensitivities and avoid them.

This method of testing for food and chemical allergy requires a spirit of dedication and a willingness to change your lifestyle to conform to the new information that results. It is very likely that you will discover that you are allergic to some of your favorite foods, and the treatment will call for you to give them up, at least temporarily. Before beginning the testing you will have to cleanse your system with a fast, which can be a difficult experience for some people. But the nuisance and the discomfort are worth it, and the payoff will be a gradual subsiding of your symptoms and a healthier and happier you.

35

The testing procedures required are:
1. removing as many possible chemical contaminants from your environment as possible;
2. fasting to clear your body; and
3. sampling foods and chemicals one at a time to determine your levels of sensitivity.

The authors do not assume responsibility for the success or failure of this program; we recommend that you explore it only under the supervision of a competent professional.

Fasting

The purpose of fasting is to rid you of as many symptoms as possible. This way your reaction to various foods will be obvious. You should obtain a thorough physical and consult your physician before beginning any fasting procedure.

Fasting, in this case, means consuming nothing but water and sea salt. The water should be pure, distilled or natural spring water that has not been stored in a plastic container.

You may be sensitive to chemicals as well as to foods. If so, it will be difficult for you accurately to assess your reactions to foods if your home is heavily loaded with odorous substances. If at all possible, plan to spend as much of the testing period as you can in an environment that is free of such odorous offenders as gas heaters and stoves, new synthetic carpeting, fresh paint, most household cleansers and soaps, and scented cosmetics and perfumes. For a more complete list of potential chemical contaminants, see the chapter titled "What Are the Sources of Allergy?"

Start by ridding your body of as much of the old offending substances and their by-products as possible. Do this by cleaning out your gastrointestinal tract. Use a laxative, like milk of magnesia or Epsom salts, or an enema.

As you withdraw from foods to which you are addicted you may experience any number of symptoms. Psychological symptoms such as mood swings and depression may accompany physiological symptoms such as stomachache, gas, headache and sore throat. Withdrawal symptoms usually begin at the end of the first or during the second day, become more troublesome on the second and third day, peak on the fourth day and then taper off. Backache and other muscle and joint aches and pains may occur on the third or fourth day and persist for a day or two. Your sense of smell and taste will probably become more acute. Your pulse rate may go either up or down, and then stabilize. This sequence of symptoms may vary greatly from person to person.

Discontinue your fast when you are free of withdrawal symptoms, when excessive hunger subsides, and when your pulse and weight stabilize. It typically requires five days to clear symptoms, but sometimes it may take seven to ten days. The average length of a fast for children is generally shorter. Arthritics and asthmatics on steroids, and persons on maintenance medications, including tranquilizers, are slower to clear.

Before beginning the fast, plan your schedule so that you can limit your activity during this important time. Your energy level may be below normal and, besides, you will want to focus as much of your attention as possible on yourself and the changes your body is undergoing.

Foods

After the fast, sample foods one at a time, three meals a day. It is important that these foods be cooked in water and seasoned only with sea salt. Otherwise it will be impossible for you to know if you are reacting to the food itself or to the seasonings.

Sample foods that you eat regularly. Eat no food more often than once every four days. Eat food from the same food family every other day. (For guidance, see the list of ''Food Families,'' pp. 132-139.)

A reaction to a food may produce a variety of symptoms. Read and reread the chapter called ''What are the Symptoms of Allergy?'' to insure that you do not overlook even mild symptoms. It is essential that you recognize each of your reactions. Otherwise, you won't receive full benefit from all your efforts. A reaction may cause a change in your pulse rate. The pulse must vary 12 to 20 points either way to be considered significant. Take your pulse by placing the second or third finger of one hand on the artery in your wrist, neck or groin area. If you take your pulse at the wrist, a slight pressure from the thumb under the wrist will help you to count each beat. Count for a full 60 seconds.

Take your pulse five minutes before eating. Eat all of the food. Then, take your pulse five, ten, twenty and forty minutes after you finish eating. Your pulse may not change for each of these readings. If your pulse varies twelve to twenty points above or below normal, it indicates a reaction to the food you are testing. For example, if your baseline pulse reading is 75, a pulse of 90 twenty minutes after eating would be significant. If your pulse continued to rise, you would know that you were reactive to the food.

Do not test a new food until you are certain that any reaction, however mild, is clear for two hours. Space meals as far apart as possible. For example, eat breakfast at 7 a.m., lunch at 1 p.m. and dinner at 7 p.m. Do not eat the next meal until your symptoms are cleared. Do not put new foods on old symptoms.

Recording the information for each test is the secret to understanding your reactions. Carefully note the time, date and food eaten. Record each pulse rate measure and all symptoms, however mild. Note the time the reaction started and the time it ended.

The following is an outline of the foods generally tested during the first week after the fast.

Day 1
Breakfast:	apples
Lunch:	potatoes
Dinner:	fish

Day 2
Breakfast:	eggs
Lunch:	chicken
Dinner:	oranges

Day 3
Breakfast:	milk and cheese
Lunch:	beef
Dinner:	pears

Day 4
Breakfast:	wheat
Lunch:	green beans or pinto beans
Dinner:	shrimp or lobster

Day 5
Breakfast:	apricots or peaches
Lunch:	broccoli or cabbage
Dinner:	pork

Day 6
Breakfast:	bananas
Lunch:	brown rice
Dinner:	lamb

Day 7   Continue eating one food at each meal, on a rotation basis. Consult your physician and discuss what you have learned during your first week of food testing.

There are several ways to clear your symptoms if they are particularly uncomfortable or if you wish to proceed with the testing.

During an allergic reaction your cells give off hydrogen ions, altering the acidity (pH) of your system. Clinically, this is called "acidosis." In order to return your body to its normal pH level, the concentration of basic ions must be increased.

An effective substance for doing this is sodium bicarbonate (baking soda). Although baking soda may relieve the troublesome symptoms it may also create an excess of sodium, so be careful if you're concerned about your salt intake. To maintain the physiological balance of other ions while correcting the highly acidic state, use an alkaline solution such as tri-alkali salts. This compound—sodium, potassium and calcium carbonates—is mixed by a pharmacist upon request in equal thirds in the total quantity desired by the individual. Tri-alkali salts do not require a prescription, but should be ordered with the approval of your physician. The usual dosage to clear a chemical or food reaction is one or two teaspoons of the mixture in eight ounces of water, followed by a second glass of water. Strong alkalinity may result in a laxative effect. It is helpful to test each carbonate separately before the pharmacist combines them, since one or two of the salts may be tolerated, but not all three.

If a reaction to a particular food develops, some other nontoxic remedies may help. *Vomiting* can be induced to help your body rid itself of a reaction to a food you've just eaten. *Laxatives*, such as Epsom salts or milk of magnesia (unflavored), are also helpful in eliminating a problem food. A warm water *enema* may bring relief. Use the same pure water that you have been drinking during the testing period.

In summary, to prepare for food testing you need to do the following:

1. Discuss fasting with your physician before you begin.
2. Purchase one serving of each food to be tested.
3. Purchase the water you will drink during the testing period, if you plan to use something other than tap water.

4. Purchase a notebook for recording your reactions.

5. Arrange your time so that you can devote yourself strictly to food testing.

The Rotation Diet is simply an extension of the testing procedures. Everything—foods, beverages and seasonings—is rotated and eaten not more often than once every four to seven days. Foods are rotated according to their food families, requiring you to eat a diversified diet that includes a wide variety of biologically unrelated foods.

Rotation and diversification prevent cross-reactions between related foods. Biologically similar foods (those in the same food family) are more likely to overload your system if they are eaten close together, before the by-products of each food are cleared from your body.

Eat all foods in the unmasked, unaddicted state on a regular schedule. Every meal becomes an acute test of whether you're sensitive to the food in question. Since no food is overused, you prevent the spread of allergy to foods you currently tolerate.

As you identify offending foods, eliminate them from your diet for three to six months. This avoidance period will give your body time to recover its ability to tolerate the food again on an occasional basis.

Even if a food has caused symptoms in the past, retest it after the three-to-six-month avoidance period. If you tolerate it in a food test, then you may safely add it to your rotation diet, in which you will eat the food not more than once every four to seven days. It is important to emphasize that once you are addicted or sensitive to a food, you can never eat it again on a daily basis without reactivating the addictive process.

In summary, remember the following principles of the rotation diet:

1. Initially, eat only one food at each meal.

2. Eat no food more often than once every four days. A single

meal of food eaten on Monday may be eaten again on Friday.
3. Skip a day between eating different foods in the same food family. For example, if peaches are eaten on Monday, apricots may be eaten on Wednesday.
4. Eat grains in the same food family no more often than once every four days. Wheat, oats and rice may be eaten with a day in between. This rule does not apply to barley and rye.
5. All fish have a common muscle. Therefore, you need to treat fish as if they were all in the same food family, and skip a day between eating any types of fish, even though they may not actually be in the same family. For instance, if you eat fish on Monday, you could eat fish of a different family on Wednesday.
6. In figuring rotation, beef and cow's milk should be spaced with a day in between. However, for testing sensitivity, eat beef and cow's milk in consecutive meals.

Chemicals

The inhalation test is an effective way for you to determine your sensitivity to common chemicals in your environment. You may have many of these chemicals on hand; others you can purchase at a drugstore.

Plan to test the following chemicals: chlorine (Clorox); phenol; formaldehyde; alcohol (ordinary rubbing alcohol); insecticide (take spray can outdoors before spraying into test jar); your favorite perfume, and cigarette smoke (test by asking a friend to smoke a cigarette in your presence).

Purchase at least four small glass jars. Place a small amount of cotton in the bottom of each jar and place five drops of chemical on each of the cotton balls. Seal the jar. Leave the substances sealed for four days before testing.

Select a definite location for all your chemical tests. For good results use a spot in which there are as few odors as possible. The room should have good ventilation and few distractions. A backporch or patio area works well. If the sniff test causes a reaction, you can then leave the odor and go inside. Sit in a comfortable chair and take your pulse. Faithfully record your pulse five minutes before each test and five, ten, twenty and forty minutes after each test. Record your pulses and other reactions, and time each test accurately.

Test only one chemical a day. Place the bottle twelve inches from your nose. Remove the top. Do not sniff the bottle. This would expose you to doses thousands of times greater than the average air levels. Record your pulse. Take another pulse at five minutes and one last pulse at ten minutes. If you react, stop testing. Record all physiological and psychological symptoms in your notebook.

It is important that you expose yourself only to the amount of the chemical suggested, at the distance recommended, and for the length of time suggested. If you experience any symptoms, stop and record results. Then begin immediately to clear yourself of the reaction.

Several non-toxic remedies will help clear you of symptoms if a reaction to a chemical develops. To clear chemical reactions, whether through exposure by inhalation or ingestion, the tri-alkali salts may be used as outlined on page 40.

Again, we want to stress the desirability of professional guidance during this or any testing procedure. The above regimen is meant only as a guideline to be used by you and your physician. The authors do not assume responsibility for the success or failure of this procedure.

The remaining chapters in this handbook will assist you in applying what you have learned. Recipes for non-toxic cosmetics and recipes to add interest to your rotation diet will follow, together with a collection of hints, lists and charts that will add to your understanding of the material we have presented so far.

Your seriousness about taking charge of your own health is demonstrated by the fact that you have read this far. We wish you luck in this endeavor and we urge you not to become discouraged. You will be rewarded by a major improvement in your health and well-being. Your self-esteem will be enhanced by undertaking and following a difficult path and—in addition to attaining a goal—you will discover that the process itself can be fun.

We wish you well on your journey to better health.

CHAPTER 8

You Can Make Your Own Cosmetics

::

COMMERCIAL COSMETICS GENERALLY CONTRI-
bute more to skin and hair *abuse* than to beauty. Every
manufactured cosmetic contains chemical preservatives, and
nearly all are made with perfumes and coloring agents.

You may find some manufacturers who have reduced the
number and intensity of common allergens in their cosmetics.
Although these may be less irritating than others, they are by
no means free from chemical contaminants.

How can you obtain cosmetics that will enhance your good
looks without exposing you to possible allergic reaction? The
answer lies in your own pantry. Many commonly available
foods can nourish your external body as well as your internal
body. If you feel creative and curious, and are willing to put a
little effort into protecting your skin and hair, experiment with
some of the unusual cosmetic recipes in this chapter.

SKIN TREATS AND TREATMENTS

SESAME MILK

Sesame milk softens, lubricates and restores the skin. It also protects against sunburn or a too-quick tan.

Ingredients: ½ cup sesame seeds; ¼ cup water
Method: **Blend seeds and water for 3 minutes. Strain.**
Use: Apply clear lotion to skin, leaving on as long as possible. Remove with warm, then cool water and blot dry.

OATMEAL LOTION

This will soften and restore roughened skin. It is especially effective on the hands.

Ingredients: 1 cup rolled oats; 6 cups water
Method: Add oats to blender to make oat flour. Mix with water and simmer 30 minutes. Strain.
Use: Wash hands. Pour small amount of lotion into palms. Apply freely and massage into skin. Do not rinse off.

OIL EMOLLIENT

These natural oils will moisturize dry skin and are especially useful on the face. You may also use them freely on dry lips, elbows, knees, legs. Any pure vegetable oil will do.

Ingredients: 1 tablespoon almond oil (for dry skin) or
1 tablespoon sesame oil (for oily skin)
Use: Open pores by applying steamy hot cloths to face. Massage oil into face at once to seal in as much moisture as possible.

MAYONNAISE MOISTURIZER

This works at least as well as any high-priced salon or commercial product.

Ingredients: 1 egg; 2 tablespoons lemon juice or vinegar; 1 cup oil
Method: Blend ingredients.
Use: Apply to face, leaving on for 30 minutes or more. Remove with warm water.

OATMEAL CLEANSER

This is a cleanser that will leave your face feeling silky.

Ingredient: 1 or 2 tablespoons oatmeal flour
Use: Splash water on face and neck. Rub oatmeal flour into wet skin. Rinse with warm, then cool water. Blot dry.

ALMOND MEAL CLEANSER

Another treat for your face.

Ingredient: 1 cup almonds
Method: Turn on blender. Pour in almonds. Grind to a fine powder. Store in airtight container.
Use: Splash water on face and rub on a handful of almond powder. Work gently into a foam. Rinse with warm, then cool water. Blot dry.

MILK CLEANSER FOR DRY SKIN

This coating removes make-up and lubricates the face.

Ingredients: 1 tablespoon whole milk; ⅛ teaspoon oil; ⅛ teaspoon honey (optional)
Method: Mix ingredients well.
Use: Apply to face. Blot off.

MILK CLEANSER FOR OILY SKIN

Ingredients: 1 or 2 teaspoons powdered milk; ¼ to ½ cup warm water

Method: Mix ingredients to a milk-like consistency.

Use: Apply to face with cotton balls. Rub gently into all areas of face. Blot dry.

MINT CLEANSER (for oily skin)

This combines cleansing power, a nice tingle and a pleasant fragrance.

Ingredients: ½ cup fresh mint leaves; 3 ice cubes

Method: Puree leaves and ice in blender. Strain.

Use: Apply clear liquid to face and allow to dry. Use throughout the day as desired, but be sure to rinse it off before retiring.

VEGETABLE CLEANSER (for oily skin)

Ingredients: 1 slice raw potato or 1 slice raw tomato

Use: Rub vegetable slice directly on face and neck. Rinse with cool water. Blot dry.

PARSLEY CLEANSER

Blackheads? Redness? Large pores? Parsley cleanser will improve these conditions.

Ingredients: ½ cup fresh parsley; 1 cup water

Method: Boil parsley for 2 minutes. Remove pot from heat. Allow to steep until lukewarm. Strain.

Use: Soak washcloth, gauze or other clean cloth in solution and apply as compress to face for 10 or 15 minutes, daily. Continue until effective.

SAGE ASTRINGENT

This is an invigorating and effective freshener.

Ingredients: ½ cup fresh sage leaves; 1 cup water
Method: Simmer sage in water for 2 minutes. Steep until lukewarm. Chill thoroughly.
Use: Moisten face freely with liquid.

MASKS

AVOCADO MASK

The most elite salons use this method; you can, too.

Ingredient: 1 ripe avocado
Method: Peel avocado. Halve. Carefully remove, clean and retain large pit, if uncracked. Puree avocado meat in blender.
Use: Cleanse face thoroughly. Spread avocado paste over face and neck. Leave on for 20 to 30 minutes. Now, take the avocado pit and use as a facial exerciser. Its unique shape and texture are well suited to this use, and will stimulate circulation. Remove mask with clear, lukewarm water. Splash face with cold water and blot dry.

PAPAYA MASK

Another fruit mask; different texture and fragrance.

Ingredient: 1 slice of fresh papaya
Use: Cleanse face. Rub face and neck well with papaya slice. Leave juice on skin for 30 minutes, reapplying as desired. Remove with warm water, rinse with cool water. Blot dry.

YEAST AND YOGURT MASK

If your face isn't a fruit fancier, these are more businesslike mask components.

Ingredients: 1 teaspoon brewer's yeast; 1 tablespoon plain yogurt

Method: Blend ingredients well.

Use: Rub mixture into face and neck. Allow to dry and remain on skin for 30 or 40 minutes. Rinse away with warm, then cool water. Use a sturdy face cloth for the final rub, then blot dry. (If undue dryness occurs, pat on a thin film of oil and blot again.)

SKIN SOFTENER

A natural way to soft and supple skin. It's effective if used regularly.

Ingredients: ½ teaspoon lemon juice (*or* rose hip powder); 1 teaspoon honey

Method: Mix ingredients thoroughly.

Use: Rub into skin, especially on hard or calloused areas. Leave on for 30 minutes. Rinse off with warm, then cool water. Blot dry.

SALLOW SKIN TONER

Ingredients: Sufficient watermelon juice, *or* 1 slice fresh papaya

Use: Apply juice (or rub slice) over desired areas of skin. Leave on as long as possible.

SKIN BLEACH

Ingredients: Unflavored yogurt or buttermilk, *or* pureed strawberries, *or* parsley juice, *or* cool tea, *or* combination of raw white potato, lemon juice and cucumber, pureed together

Use:	Apply to dark or blotchy areas of skin and leave on for at least 30 minutes, daily.

SUNSCREEN & SKIN AID

PABA stands for para-aminobenzoic acid, an element of the vitamin B complex. This nutrient will provide full protection from the harmful band of the sunlight spectrum.

Ingredients:	1 tablespoon PABA Cream, *or* PABA tablets, powdered and mixed with oil
Use:	Apply before exposing skin to sunlight. It will be effective for about 2 hours of heavy exercise, or for about 1 hour if applied after swimming.

Another nutrient that is useful in easing sunburn is vitamin E, frequently available as a cream or lotion. Make sure that you buy the one *without* perfume or other additives. The ultimate in portable sunscreen is a vitamin E capsule, which can be punctured to provide pure vitamin E on the spot.

BATHS

OIL BATH

This is beneficial for the skin, and it feels good, too. There's a good reason why "anointing the body with oil" is an ancient ritual of honor and respect.

Ingredient:	1 or 2 cups oil (Dry skin: almond, olive or peanut oil; oily skin: sesame, sunflower or corn oil; wheat germ oil is good for both types.)
Method:	Heat to desired degree of warmth (110° to 130° F, not hot).
Use:	Carefully massage oil into skin over your entire

body. Start with the feet and work upwards, slowly, with firm massage pressure. When body is well coated, gently run the edge of your hand up the body, to remove excess. (Wipe hand on paper towel frequently.) When excess oil has been removed, immerse your body in a tub of water, warm enough to dissolve remaining oil. Massage the entire body under water. Then proceed with usual bath routine.

VINEGAR BATH

Ingredient: ¼ cup vinegar
Method: Add to bath water.
Regular use of alkaline soap can cause drying and scaling of the skin. This will counteract the alkalinity and prevent or ease such scaling.

BODY SCOUR

Salt provides an invigorating body scour that increases circulation, draws off impurities, sloughs off dead skin, and leaves the body feeling alive and glowing.

Ingredient: 1 or 2 cups sea salt (ordinary table salt is not as coarse and much less effective)
Use: Wet body in shower or bath. Pour sea salt into your cupped hand and work upward, beginning with toes, heels, feet, ankles. Continue to gently rub sea salt into your moistened skin (avoiding cut, bruised or recently shaved areas) until entire body has been massaged. Allow salt to cling until water evaporates. (For tender facial skin, use salt moistened with a small amount of oil.) Proceed with usual bath.

SHAMPOOS AND RINSES

OILY HAIR SHAMPOO

Shampoo is a Hindu word that originally meant to touch or massage. To get the full benefit from any kind of shampoo, don't forget to massage well and long while you apply it.

Ingredients: 1 whole egg; ½ teaspoon vinegar; 1 tablespoon lemon juice; 1 ounce pure castile.

Method: Blend ingredients well, by hand or in blender.

Use: Wet hair thoroughly, apply shampoo, massage, and rinse. A second application, using much less shampoo, will insure thorough cleansing.

VINEGAR RINSE

The hair is protected by a natural acidic mantle that is destroyed by virtually any shampoo. This will ensure correct pH balance.

Ingredients: 1 teaspoon vinegar; 1 cup water

Method: Mix ingredients.

Use: After thoroughly rinsing shampooed hair, apply the vinegar rinse. Work into scalp thoroughly. Allow to remain 1 or 2 minutes, then rinse in clear warm water.

HERBAL RINSE

Ingredients: ⅛ cup *each* of camomile and raspberry leaves; ½ cup rosemary leaves; 3 cups water. (If hair is very oily, add ⅛ cup dried witch hazel.)

Method: Combine ingredients and simmer for 10 minutes. Steep until lukewarm. Strain.

Use: After shampoo, massage 2 tablespoons of Herbal Rinse into hair. Leave on for 5 minutes, then rinse thoroughly.

EGG CONDITIONER

Ingredient: 1 or 2 egg yolks
Method: Beat yolks with small amount of water.
Use: Dry hair thoroughly. Brush well. Coat every strand of hair and every area of scalp with yolk mixture, using slow, firm, circular motion. Wrap towel around head and allow solution to remain on hair and scalp for 30 minutes. Rinse out thoroughly with warm water. Rinse again with cool water.

AVOCADO CONDITIONER

Ingredient: 1 ripe avocado
Method: Mash well.
Use: Massage into hair and scalp for 5 minutes. Wrap hair in towel and leave avocado in contact with hair for 1 hour. Rinse out and shampoo in usual manner.

OIL CONDITIONER

These oils are the source of fatty acids, which are essential to the well-nourished body.

Ingredient: 1 cup of oil (castor, almond, sesame or similar oil).
Method: Heat enough oil to cover entire scalp.
Use: Gently comb oil into hair, until all of the hair is well coated. Comb through each strand several times. Wrap one or two towels around your head to create and retain as much scalp heat as possible. (This will help the oil to penetrate the hair.) Leave towels on for at least 1 hour, then proceed with usual shampoo and rinse.

MAYONNAISE CONDITIONER

This is a different consistency than the Egg Conditioner, and the addition of vinegar helps to restore the natural acid balance of the hair.

Ingredients: 2 egg yolks; 2 tablespoons vinegar; 1 cup oil
Method: Blend ingredients at high speed in blender.
Use: Massage well into hair and scalp. Leave in contact for 1 hour, then shampoo and rinse.

BRIGHT AND SHINY CONDITIONER

For gleaming, radiant, glossy hair.

Ingredients: 1 cup honey; 1 or 2 cups olive oil
Method: Shake ingredients together in a covered jar until they are well mixed. Steep for 2 days before using. Shake again just before use.
Use: Dry hair well. Apply mixture to one section of scalp at a time, massaging thoroughly into hair and scalp. Generate and retain scalp heat by covering head with 1 or 2 towels. Leave towels in place for 1 hour. Shampoo as usual.

HAIR COLOR

These natural vegetable and plant coloring agents result in a very slight tint. The shades will vary with each person because of individual body chemistry.

BLONDE RINSE

Ingredients: 1 cup camomile loose tea; 2 cups water.
Method: Simmer tea in water for 30 minutes. Allow to cool, then strain out leaves.
Use: Shampoo hair as usual. Rinse well in clear, warm

water. Place your head over a bowl and pour tea through your hair several times. Gently comb hair and pour tea through hair again to ensure complete coverage. Squeeze out excess moisture (do *not* rinse) and towel dry. For best results, dry your golden hair in the sunlight.

RHUBARB ROOT LIGHTENER

Ingredients: ½ cup rhubarb root; 3 cups water

Method: Simmer rhubarb in water, uncovered, for 30 minutes. Steep mixture overnight, then strain out solids.

Use: Shampoo as usual. Towel dry hair. Pour liquid lightener through hair repeatedly, catching runoff in a bowl beneath your head. The light color will intensify if you allow your hair to dry in the sun.

SAGE DARKENER

Ingredients: ½ cup dried sage; 2 cups water

Method: Simmer sage in water for 30 minutes. Steep for 4 hours and strain.

Use: Wash hair. Pour liquid darkener through hair several times. Do not rinse. Towel dry.

OTHER HAIR CARE PREPARATIONS

LEMON HAIR SPRAY

This use of lemon is a less-than-perfect hair spray, but an acceptable substitute for commercial, chemically loaded products. It may be drying if used frequently, resulting in brittle hair.

Ingredients: 1 lemon; 1 cup water

Method: Chop lemon. Cover with water and boil until only half the original quantity of liquid remains. Cool. Strain lemon liquid through a thin cloth or a fine mesh strainer. (If the residue is too thick, add some water and mix well.) Store in a fine-spray dispenser bottle and refrigerate. EMERGENCY USE: When you have an important engagement, a flyaway hair problem, and insufficient time to create the above, squeeze lemon juice into palm of your hand and pat on unruly hair.

HAIR SETTING LOTION

This mixture works better with normal or oily hair than it does on dry hair. You'll discover the right amount of collagen for *your* hair with some experimentation. Too much and your hair will appear dry from the coating; too little and you won't notice the benefit.

Ingredients: ¼ to ¾ teaspoons liquid predigested collagen protein (obtainable from health food stores); 1 cup water; and
FOR BRUNETTES: 1 tablespoon rosemary
FOR BLONDES: 1 tablespoon camomile
ESPECIALLY FOR DRY HAIR: ⅛ teaspoon oil

Method: Steep herb in boiling water. Cool to lukewarm. Blend in protein. (Add oil for dry hair.)

Use: Massage into hair thoroughly, and allow hair to set.

OTHER COSMETIC SUBSTITUTES AND AIDS

ALOE VERA CURE-ALL

Aloe Vera is a cactus plant with properties that ease many ailments. Burns, sunburn, flaky skin, dry skin and dandruff are just a few of the unwelcome conditions that it can aid. You can get your own aloe vera cactus plant from most nurseries, or buy the gel from a health food store, but be sure you don't buy a version that has a preservative in it.

Ingredient: Aloe vera leaf or gel

Use: Apply directly on affected area.

FENNEL EYEWASH

For inflamed eyelids or eyes that are watering to excess.

Ingredients: 1 teaspoon dried fennel, *or* ⅓ cup fresh fennel; 1 cup water

Method: Boil fennel in water for 10 minutes. Steep until the mixture is lukewarm. Strain.

Use: Put 2 drops into open eye with eye dropper and blink a few times. Close eyes and gently move them from side to side. Another method of application is to soak compresses in fennel tea and place over eyelids.

NAIL COLORING

All commercial nail polish is toxic. This is an ancient cosmetic, used successfully since the time of the Pharaohs. This natural method is a lot of trouble, but the result lasts a long time. Apply carefully; if the skin adjacent to the nail gets color on it, the color will be difficult to remove. The pink part of the nail will turn out darker than the white half moon. Henna leaves can usually be found in beauty supply shops or salons.

Ingredients: ¼ teaspoon dried henna leaves, powdered; water

Method: Mix henna powder with only enough water to make a thick paste.

Use: Rub paste into nails. Allow to dry for at least 1 hour. For a deeper color, dry with heat, using your hair dryer, for 15 to 30 minutes. Buff to the pale red-orange shade you prefer.

LAVENDER COLOGNE

For a fresh, old fashioned fragrance, this can't be matched by anything store-bought.

Ingredients: 2 drops pure lavender oil; ¼ teaspoon water

Method: Mix water and oil thoroughly.

Use: Apply freely to freshly-washed underarm, and body heat-producing areas.

CHAPTER NINE

How You Can Eat Well And Safely

∷∷∷

NOW THAT YOU KNOW SOMETHING ABOUT WHAT allergies are, how they work, how to discover if you have them, and—if you do—how to avoid allergy-producing substances, where do you go from here?

One of the principal sources of allergens may be the food you eat. To help you avoid the foods to which you are sensitive, and to aid in both testing and treating your food allergies, the authors have assembled (in some cases invented) and tested a collection of unusual recipes.

By and large, these dishes are simple to prepare; they call for easily available ingredients and they may intrigue you with their uncommon combinations of foods. They will add creativity and delight to the process of being careful about what you and your family eat.

Most important, they have been designed to use ingredients from a *minimal* number of food families, so that if you are trying the Rotation Diet to discover your own allergic food reactions, these recipes will not blur the results.

Read through the recipes and try a few that interest you. You'll be delighted with the results.

FRUIT

AMBROSIA

3 oranges   1 tablespoon fresh lemon juice
1 medium grapefruit   1 cup grated coconut
8 tablespoons honey

Peel oranges and grapefruit. Divide into sections and add honey and lemon juice. Toss with coconut and serve well chilled.

APPLE AND CARROT SALAD

5 medium youngish carrots   1 tablespoon cider vinegar or
2 firm apples   2 tablespoons apple juice

Grate carrots. Cut apples into small cubes. Toss with vinegar or apple juice. Chill well before serving.

PINEAPPLE-PAPAYA PERFECTION

½ fresh pineapple   ½ fresh papaya

Remove top and bottom of pineapple. (The top, if placed cut side down in a bowl of water, will sprout roots and in time will give you a durable, lovely house plant!) Score the pineapple in a downward spiral with the point of a sharp knife to remove the eyes. Peel and cube. Peel papaya, dice and toss with pineapple for an unusual taste combination.

BERRY SALAD

1 cup fresh strawberries   (Try substituting blackberries or
1 cup fresh blueberries   raspberries for the strawberries
                                                 and huckleberries or cranberries
                                                 for the blueberries)

Hull, clean and slice strawberries. Crush blueberries. Thin slightly with water and serve, chilled, layered over strawberries.

WALDORF SALAD

1 cup chopped cashews   ¼ cup apple juice
2 apples (crisp fall apples are
  best)

Chop cashews. Dice apples and combine with cashews and apple juice. Serve chilled. (If the apples are brightly colored, leave unpeeled when dicing. Apples should be tart.) The original version included thinly sliced celery, homemade mayonnaise flavored with mustard, and English walnuts instead of cashews.

MELON MAGIC

Cantaloupe, honeydew, casaba
or any other fresh, ripe melon
in season.

Halve melon. Use melon-baller to scoop out pulp. (If you don't have one, a demitasse spoon will serve, or you can cut out pulp and dice into small cubes.) Place melon balls into cellophane bag and freeze. Serve without syrup.

BANANA PANCAKES

2 ripe bananas
2 eggs
1 teaspoon honey

Blend all ingredients together until smooth. Spoon onto hot, lightly greased griddle. Turn once and serve golden brown.

APPLE OR PEAR SAUCE

Fresh, firm apples or pears   *Cinnamon (optional)*

Quarter fruit, removing core and seeds. Steam until tender. Puree in blender. Serve hot or cold.

BAKED APPLE SLICES

1 cup sliced apples   *½ cup maple syrup*
1 cup chopped nuts (optional)

Preheat oven to 350° F. Combine apple slices and nuts in baking pan. Pour maple syrup over apples and mix lightly. Bake for 20 minutes, or until apples are tender. Baste with syrup occasionally.

APRICOT AMAZEMENTS

1 cup dried apricots   *½ cup honey*
1 cup almonds

Cover apricots with water and soak overnight. Chop half the almonds and grind the other half. Dice apricots; add honey and chopped almonds. Cook slowly over low heat until thick, *stirring constantly*. Cool, shape into small balls and roll them in the ground almonds. Chill thoroughly.

FRUIT STEW

Dried fruits

Barely cover with water and soak overnight. Heat gently until tender and serve either warm or cold.

DRIED FRUIT JAM

Dried fruits   *honey*

Soak fruit in water for at least 3 hours. Drain and puree in blender. Slowly add honey until the jam is the desired consistency and sweetness.

BERRY JAMBOREE

4 cups berries   *2 cups honey*

Puree berries and honey in blender. Boil rapidly over high heat, stirring until very thick. Immediately ladle into hot, sterile jars. Seal. Yield: 2 pints.

APPLE BUTTER

4 pounds apples   *Optional: 1 teaspoon cinnamon*
2 cups apple juice   *1 teaspoon ground*
1 cup honey   *cloves*
                              ½ teaspoon allspice

Peel and core apples. Puree with other ingredients. Cook rapidly until thick. Pour while hot into sterile jars, sealing them at once. Yield: 5 pints.

PINEAPPLE FREEZE

6 eggs   *4 cups fresh pineapple*
1¼ cups honey   *1 cup ice water*

Separate eggs. Beat egg whites until stiff. In a separate bowl, blend yolks with honey. Fold yolk mixture into whites. Puree pineapple in blender and add water. Combine pineapple with egg mixture and freeze.

WATERMELON ICE

1 quart watermelon chunks   Juice of one lemon
½ cup honey

Seed watermelon. Mix all ingredients and steep overnight. Blend at low speed, freeze until partially solid then blend again at high speed. Freeze. (If frozen in ice cube trays with a stick in each cube, you'll produce watermelon ice popsicles.)

ORANGE SHERBET

The French call it *sorbet*, but it is one of the earliest known desserts, originally from the Middle East. It probably began as a sweetened fruit drink chilled with snow.

6 cups fresh or frozen orange   4 cups honey
  juice   3 cups water
2 tablespoons orange rind

Mix all ingredients and freeze. (Experiment with other fruits; pear is absolutely unique).

FRUIT SLUSH UPPER

This is a real pick-me-up: a zippy way to start the day or a marvelous lift for the late afternoon blahs.

½ fresh pineapple   2 cups orange juice
2 bananas

Chop pineapple and freeze. Puree bananas and freeze in ice cube tray. Puree frozen fruits with orange juice.

HOT APPLE HONEY

2 cups apple juice   2 teaspoons honey

Mix. Heat slowly until honey is dissolved. Serve warm.

LEMONADE

7 lemons (or 10 limes)   3 cups water
1/4 cup honey

Juice lemons or limes. Mix with honey. Add water and stir vigorously. Serve over ice.

SHAM-PAGNE

2 lemons (or 4 limes)   6 ounces Perrier water
1/4 cup apple juice   2 thin slices lemon

Squeeze citrus and mix thoroughly with apple juice. Chill. When ready to serve, pour over ice; add Perrier for sparkle and float lemon slices.

WINE

20 pounds of grapes, berries or   5 quarts water
      other fresh fruit   10 cups raw sugar

Mash fruit in ceramic bowl. (Don't use a metal container; it will affect the taste). Boil water and add to fruit. Cover well and allow to stand for 3 days. Strain through cheese-cloth and add raw sugar. Return to jar and cover tightly. Let mixture stand until fermentation has ceased. Remove scum and strain juice. Bottle in sterile containers and seal.

VEGETABLES

Steamed vegetables can be interesting. Remember not to steam too long: *al dente* (which in Italian means that you need to use your teeth) not only preserves nutrients but is a more rewarding way to eat. You can steam vegetables by bringing ¼ cup of water to a boil, adding vegetables and simmering in a well-covered pan until tender. Another method is to use a steamer basket to hold the vegetables above the water inside a covered pan.

CHARD PIE

This is surprisingly tasty, and you can substitute other mild greens for chard.

50 leaves chard	*3 eggs*
1 medium onion	*1 cup natural cheese, grated*

Preheat oven to 350° F. Clean chard well in running water. Chop onion and steam in oven-proof pan for 3 minutes. Add chard and steam until wilted. Beat eggs and stir into vegetable mixture. Sprinkle with grated cheese and bake for 15 minutes.

WILTED SPINACH

1 pound spinach	*1 tablespoon olive or other oil*
½ cup cashews	

Clean spinach well. Chop cashews and sauté in oil until golden. Add spinach and cook 2 to 3 minutes.

PLURAL SQUASH CASSEROLE

If you're tired of squash, this dish will provide relief. Combining different varieties adds color and offers a different taste. It is a good main dish.

1 butternut or acorn squash
1 yellow squash
1 white squash
¼ cup water
1½ cups cheese, grated

Peel and slice butternut squash. Slice other squash, removing large seeds. Boil water and add squash slices. Sprinkle with grated cheese and cook 8 to 12 minutes. Don't overcook; the squash will be more satisfying if it is still somewhat firm, not limp.

BAKED SQUASH

1 butternut or acorn squash
2 tablespoons butter

2 teaspoons raw brown sugar
1 teaspoon ground cinnamon (optional)

Preheat oven to 350° F. Halve squash, removing large seeds. Dot with butter and sprinkle with brown sugar and cinnamon. Bake for 20 minutes or until tender. (This is an unusual breakfast dish, nourishing and satisfying.)

PINEAPPLE AND SQUASH

½ fresh pineapple
2 acorn or butternut squash

3 tablespoons butter

Preheat oven to 350° F. Peel pineapple and dice. Layer with squash in small loaf pan with pineapple on top. Dot with butter and bake for 30 minutes. (Another eye-opening breakfast dish.)

APPLE CARROT GLAZE

2 cups cooked carrots, sliced   3 tablespoons raw brown sugar
¼ cup applesauce   5 teaspoons butter

Preheat oven to 350° F. Combine all ingredients in ovenproof dish. Cover and bake for 15 minutes.

STUFFED EGGPLANT

1 eggplant   Grated mozzarella or
¼ green pepper   parmesan cheese
2 tablespoons lemon juice

Preheat oven to 350° F. Cut eggplant in half and scoop out flesh. Chop into cubes and steam for about 4 minutes. Seed and chop pepper. Add to eggplant and mix with lemon juice. Fill shells with mixture and sprinkle with grated cheese. Bake for 20 minutes or until tender.

RHUBARB REWARD

2 cups rhubarb   2 teaspoons cinnamon
½ cup honey

Preheat oven to 300° F. Slice rhubarb and layer into oiled baking dish, alternating with layers of honey. Sprinkle with cinnamon. Bake until rhubarb is red, about 25 minutes.

FRIED OKRA

1 pound okra
½ cup rice flour
4 tablespoons rice oil

Cut okra and shake with flour in paper bag until well coated.

Heat oil in skillet and fry okra, stirring frequently, for 10 to 15 minutes.

BAKED BEETS

3 beets, cooked   *2 tablespoons flour*
¼ cup honey   *¼ teaspoon salt (optional)*
½ cup orange juice

Preheat oven to 350° F. Slice beets, arrange in oiled baking dish. Combine remaining ingredients and pour over beets. Cover and bake for 30 minutes.

LENTIL SOUP

8 leeks (optional)   *3 cups water*
1 cup lentils   *¼ teaspoon salt*

Chop leeks. Boil water and add leeks and lentils. Simmer one hour or until done, adding water as needed.

SWEET POTATO AND PINEAPPLE

Another uncommonly good breakfast item.

1 large sweet potato   *½ fresh pineapple*

Peel both ingredients and chop. Mix and steam until tender.

SWEET POTATO PUDDING

A good dessert and a great day-starter.

2 tablespoons boiling water   *2 tablespoons honey*
¼ cup raisins   *½ cup orange juice*
1 large sweet potato   *¼ teaspoon grated orange rind*

Boil water and pour 2 tablespoons over raisins. Peel and dice sweet potato and steam until tender. Mix with honey, raisins, juice and rind. Beat well.

SWEET POTATO BREAD

1 cup sweet potato	*½ cup oil*
1¾ cup flour	*2 eggs*
1½ cups raw sugar	*½ cup nuts*
1 teaspoon cinnamon	*⅓ cup water*
¼ teaspoon salt	

Preheat oven to 350° F. Peel, dice, steam, and mash sweet potato. Sift together flour, sugar, cinnamon and salt. Add mixture to sweet potatoes, stirring in oil and water. Beat in eggs and add nuts. Mixture will fill two small greased loaf pans or one standard-size loaf pan. Bake for 1 hour. Remove from pans immediately.

POTATO PANCAKES

4 large potatoes	*2 tablespoons potato starch*
1 egg	

Peel and grate potatoes. Beat egg gently with fork and add to potatoes. Stir in starch and mix well. Spoon mixture onto greased griddle at low temperature. Cook until brown around edges and turn once with spatula. (A favorite version of this dish adds grated onion to the potato mixture. Pancakes will be crisper if spooned onto griddle thinly.)

ROSTI POTATOES

A company dish!

3 medium potatoes	*½ cup onion, diced*
¼ cup oil or butter	*1¼ teaspoon salt*

Scrub potatoes and steam until tender. Drain and chill thoroughly. Peel and shred or grate coarsely. Melt butter in skillet and add onion, cooking until tender, about 5 minutes. Add potatoes and salt. Cook for 15 minutes, turning frequently Press mixture into flat cake with spatula, sprinkle with hot water and cover. Cook over low heat until crusty.

NOT-QUITE-FRENCH FRIES

An especially good recipe if you prefer not to serve fried foods.

4 medium potatoes	¼ cup soy oil (or other oil)
1 teaspoon salt	

Preheat oven to 400° F. Peel and slice potatoes. Pour oil into 9″ × 13″ pan. Coat slices with oil and arrange in pan. Bake for 30 to 40 minutes. Sprinkle with salt.

HOT POTATO SALAD

3 medium potatoes	¼ cup grape vinegar (wine vin-
1 onion	egar is okay, but watch for additives).

Peel and chop potatoes into small pieces. Dice onions and toss with 1 tablespoon vinegar, adding to potatoes. Steam until tender and stir in remaining vinegar. Serve at once.

POTATO BRIOCHE

A company treat. In the unlikely event that any are left, they are fine reheated.

1 cup leftover mashed potatoes	¼ cup potato starch
2 egg yolks	

Preheat oven to 350° F. Mix two-thirds of mashed potatoes with 1 egg yolk. Dust pastry board with starch and flatten mixture to 1-inch thickness. Cut out rounds with cookie cutter. These will become brioche bases. Make a thumb depression in each round and use remaining one-third of potato mixture to fashion 1-inch diameter balls. Place on top of brioche base. Brush all over with remaining egg yolk and bake until brown and glossy.

STUFFED TOMATOES

4 eggs
3 celery stalks

4 tomatoes

Hard-boil eggs. Chop celery. Scoop out insides of tomatoes, turn upside down, remove pulp and drain pulp for 2 hours. Chop hard-boiled eggs with half of tomato pulp and mix with celery. Stuff mixture into tomato shells and chill.

ZESTY ZUCCHINI

1 zucchini
2 stalks celery
1 green pepper
2 tomatoes

1 red pepper, banana pepper
or chili pepper
4 tablespoons tomato purée

Chop zucchini and steam for 3 minutes. Chop other ingredients and mix with zucchini. Marinate in tomato puree overnight. Serve cold.

CARROT SALAD

1 cup carrots
¼ cup grapefruit sections

¼ cup grapefruit juice

Grate carrots and toss with fruit and juice. Serve cold.

SUPER SPINACH

1 cup fresh spinach
1 tablespoon oil
1 clove garlic, crushed

3 tablespoons lemon juice
1 cup crushed filberts

Wash spinach well in cold water and tear into bite-sized pieces. Toss lightly with oil. Add garlic, lemon juice and nuts. Toss, chill for an hour, toss again and serve.

THREE SLAWS

Almost any salad made primarily with shredded raw cabbage is considered cole slaw. You can vary the taste significantly by adding a single chopped fruit and moistening with the juice of that fruit.

Three suggestions:

Chopped grapefruit and grapefruit juice; chopped apple and apple juice or cider vinegar; chopped pineapple and pineapple juice. In each case, toss and serve chilled. Experiment!

THREE BEAN SALAD

¼ cup dried pinto beans
1 cup fresh green beans

½ cup fresh green peas
¾ cup vinegar

Soak pinto beans overnight in 2 cups of water. Simmer until done, about 4 hours. Steam cut green beans and peas. Mix beans together with vinegar and marinate 12 hours. Serve chilled.

PRETTY PICKLES

1 gallon cucumbers	*2 tablespoons honey*
16 garlic cloves	*2 quarts vinegar*
6 sprigs fresh dill	*4 quart jars with tight lids*
2 teaspoons salt	

Slice or quarter cucumbers. Combine with other ingredients and bring to a boil. Ladle into hot, sterile quart jars. Seal.

FISH

POACHED FISH

Most gourmets prefer the subtle taste of poached fish. Bring about an inch of water to the boiling point in a shallow pan. Slip fish into water, cover, and cook gently 5 to 7 minutes. Remove with slotted spatula or spoon.

FRIED FISH

Sprinkle fish with lemon juice or water. Coat with any of the following:

ground cashews or other nuts;   *arrowroot starch; ground oats.*
sesame seeds; rice or corn flour;

Fry in oil until crisp.

BROILED FISH

1 fresh fish fillet
2 tablespoons lemon juice
1 lemon

Preheat broiler. Dip fish into lemon juice. Thinly slice lemon and arrange slices in bottom of baking dish, placing fish on top. Broil about 5 minutes or until fish is flaky.

BAKED FISH

2 *medium onions*   *1 pound fresh fish fillet*
2 *tomatoes*

Preheat oven to 400° F. Peel and slice onion. Steam for 5 to 8 minutes, until tender. Puree tomatoes. Arrange half of the onion slices in a baking dish, with fish on top. Place remaining onion slices over fish and pour tomato puree over fish and onions. Bake for 25 minutes.

SESAME FISH

2 *tablespoons sesame seeds*   *1 pound fresh fish fillets*
3 *leeks or green onions*   *¼ cup tamari or soy sauce*

Preheat broiler. Toast sesame seeds. Chop leeks. Cut fish into pieces, dipping each chunk into tamari, then rolling in seeds to coat. Broil 3 to 4 minutes and serve with tamari for seasoning.

SKILLET FISH

⅛ teaspoon chili pepper   *1½ pounds cooked fish (or*
1 *small cauliflower*   *1 large can tuna)*
2 *tablespoons onion*

Preheat oven to 400° F. Chop chili pepper or substitute cayenne pepper. Boil and mash cauliflower. Mince onion. Combine all ingredients and shape into patties. Bake 8 minutes or fry until golden brown.

FISH AMANDINE

1 fresh fish fillet   *¹/₄ cup almonds*
4 tablespoons butter

Broil fish. Melt butter and sauté slivered almonds until lightly browned. Sprinkle over fish and serve at once.

FILLET SAUTÉ

4 tablespoons butter   *¹/₂ cup fresh mushrooms*
1 fresh fish fillet

Melt butter. Sauté fish, turning once. Clean and mince mushrooms. Remove fish (keeping it warm) and sauté mushrooms for 2 minutes. Pour over fish and serve.

CHICKEN

Like fish, chicken can be coated with any of the following: ground cashews or other nuts; sesame seeds; rice or corn flour; arrowroot starch; ground oats. Dip chicken pieces in water and roll in coating you have chosen. Fry in oil or bake at 350° for 45 minutes.

CHICKEN AND RICE

¹/₂ cup onion   *1 cup chicken (boned)*
3 tablespoons butter   *1 cup cooked rice*

Dice onion and sauté in butter. Dice chicken. Add rice to sautéed onion and turn with spatula as it starts to brown. Add chicken and cook until chicken is firm and white.

CHICKEN AND AVOCADO SALAD

1 medium avocado   *¼ cooked chicken*

Peel avocado and cut into small pieces. Remove skin and dice chicken. Combine and chill.

CHICKEN SALAD

1 chicken   *2 cups cashews or other nuts*
4 apples   *½ cup apple juice*

Steam chicken until tender. Bone and cut meat into bite-sized pieces. Chop apples and add to chicken. Add nut and apple juice. Chill thoroughly and serve cold.

CHICKEN AND POTATO DUMPLINGS

1 chicken   *½ cup potato starch*
3 potatoes   *1½ teaspoons salt*
1 egg   *4 cups chicken broth*

Cover chicken with water and simmer until tender, about 45 minutes. Remove, cool, bone and chop. Steam potatoes. Chill thoroughly. Peel and grate. Mix potatoes with egg, starch and salt. Beat until fluffy. Shape potato mixture into small balls and drop into hot chicken broth. Cook covered for about 4 minutes. Add chopped chicken and simmer for another 2 to 4 minutes.

CHICKEN AND WHEAT DUMPLINGS

1½ cups whole wheat flour   *3 tablespoons oil*
¾ teaspoon salt   *¾ cup milk or water*
2 teaspoons baking powder   *1 cooked chicken*

Combine flour, salt and baking powder. Add oil, then stir

in liquid. Boil chicken until hot—5 to 10 minutes. Drop dumplings by spoonful into same boiling broth. Cook uncovered for 10 minutes. Cover and cook for another 10 minutes.

CHICKEN AND RICE SOUP

1 stewed chicken
4 cups chicken broth
1 cup cooked rice

1 cup celery
½ cup onion

Bone and dice chicken. Simmer broth in quart pot, adding rice. Chop celery and onion; add to broth. Simmer for 20 minutes.

GAME

FRIED VENISON

1 pound venison
½ cup rice flour

1 cup rice oil

Dip venison in water, shake, and roll in flour. Fry in hot oil, turning once.

DEER STEAKS

1 pound deer steak
8 tablespoons butter or oil

½ cup onion
2 tablespoons vinegar

Cut meat into serving pieces and brown in 5 tablespoons butter. Mince onion and sauté in separate pan in remaining butter. Combine onions and meat and simmer 25 minutes, stirring occasionally. Add vinegar and simmer 5 minutes more.

VENISON CHILI

1 pound ground venison	½ cup green pepper
1 onion	2 cups hot water
2 tablespoons chili powder or chopped red pepper	2 teaspoons salt

Brown meat well. Chop onion. Mix all ingredients and simmer 30 minutes or longer. Season to taste, cool, then reheat and serve.

RABBIT STEW

1 rabbit	1 bay leaf
1 quart vinegar	1 onion
1 quart water	1 teaspoon salt

Soak rabbit in vinegar and water overnight in refrigerator. Discard liquid. Cover rabbit with fresh water, add other ingredients and simmer over low heat until tender.

OTHER MEATS

CHEESY LAMB CHOPS

4 lamb chops	4 slices cheese
1 onion	

Broil chops about 7 minutes on each side. Thinly slice onion. Place sliced onion on each chop, then cover with cheese slice. Broil until cheese melts, about 2 minutes more.

LIVER DUMPLINGS

1 pound liver	5 cups beef broth
1 tablespoon butter	2 eggs
1 onion	Pepper to taste
1 cup dried bread crumbs	1 tablespoon salt
1 cup flour	

Simmer liver in water for 30 minutes. Remove membrane and ducts. Grind or mince liver. Mince onion and sauté in butter, adding bread crumbs, salt and pepper. Add enough flour to beaten eggs to make a stiff batter. Boil broth, dropping batter from tablespoon into broth. Cover well and cook for 30 minutes.

MEAT STEW

2 pounds stew meat (lamb or beef)	2 teaspoons salt
2 potatoes	½ teaspoon pepper
1 tablespoon potato starch	½ cup water

Cut meat into serving portions, removing excess fat. Brown and then simmer covered for 30 minutes. Cut potatoes into chunks or slices. Add to meat and simmer another 30 minutes. Dissolve starch in small amount of cold water; add to stew to thicken. Season well, stir and serve.

PORK

PORK ROAST

1 pork roast	1 cup apple juice

Preheat oven to 325° F. Brown roast well. Place in roasting dish. Pour juice over roast and cook until very well done—at least 30 minutes per pound.

SKILLET PORK CASSEROLE

4 pork chops	1 pineapple
1 green pepper	½ cup tomato purée
2 tomatoes	

Dice pork, green pepper, tomatoes, and pineapple. Heat small amount of pork fat, brown pork and pepper. Add pineapple, tomatoes and tomato puree. Simmer 30 minutes or until pork is completely cooked. Serve hot or cold.

SWEET AND SOUR PORK

2 pork chops	2 cups pineapple chunks
¼ cup soy flour	¼ cup honey
½ cup soy oil	2 teaspoons soy sauce or tamari

Dice pork, roll in flour and brown well in oil over medium heat, turning frequently. Puree half of pineapple in blender. Mix pureed pineapple with honey, soy sauce and remaining cup of pineapple chunks. Cook until smooth and thick, stirring frequently. Pour over browned pork and serve.

BREADED PORK CHOPS

1 cup nuts	2 pork chops

Preheat oven to 350° F. Grind nuts in blender. Dip chops in water, shake and roll in nuts. Bake for 45 minutes or until very well done.

SAUSAGE PATTIES

1 pound ground pork	⅛ teaspoon sage
1 teaspoon salt	¼ teaspoon thyme
⅛ teaspoon pepper	

Mix ingredients, shaping into small cakes. Thoroughly fry until meat is white inside and crispy brown outside.

PEPPER AND PORK

¼ cup onion   1 pound ground pork
4 medium green or red bell   1 cup stewed tomatoes
  peppers

Preheat oven to 350° F. Peel and chop onion. Remove stems and seeds from peppers. Steam peppers 3 to 5 minutes. Combine pork and onion and brown well. Add tomatoes and simmer 5 minutes. Stuff peppers with meat mixture and bake for 25 minutes, until very well done.

PORK AND FRUIT

Pork combines surprisingly well with fruit, especially if the fruit is tart.

4 green bell peppers   1 pound ground pork
2 fresh pears or apples   ½ cup grated cheese

Preheat oven to 350° F. Remove pepper stems and cut each pepper in half vertically. Remove seeds. Steam peppers for 3 to 5 minutes. Mince fruit and combine with meat. Brown well. Stuff peppers with meat mixture and sprinkle with grated cheese. Bake for 15 minutes.

PORK AND SQUASH

2 acorn or butternut squash   ¼ cup molasses
1 pound ground pork

Preheat broiler. Halve squash and steam until tender. Brown pork thoroughly. Spread squash with molasses and fill halves with meat. Brown under broiler and serve at once.

EGGS

BASIC EGGS

For a *Not-Quite-Fried Egg*, cover bottom of frying pan with water and heat to boiling point. Break egg over center of skillet, cook to desired doneness and turn once. *Scrambled Eggs* without oil can be cooked in a similar manner: break egg and beat slightly with a fork, pour into center of skillet just covered with boiling water. Reduce heat; slowly stir and turn constantly until water has evaporated. *Poached Eggs* call for about 1 inch of water in a shallow pan. Bring water to a boil and reduce heat to simmer. Break each egg into saucer and quickly, smoothly, slip into water. Cook covered for 3 to 5 minutes. Lift out of pan with slotted spatula or spoon. Drain well.

SOUFFLÉ

4 eggs
3 tablespoons butter

Preheat oven to 350° F. Chill eggs and separate yolks from whites. Let stand at room temperature for 1 hour. Beat yolks until light and thick. Beat whites until stiff. Fold yolks into whites slowly. Melt butter in oven-proof pan and pour in egg mixture. Cook over low heat for 3 minutes without stirring, then bake for 15 minutes. (This recipe dresses up any meal. Or it will serve you well when you're tired of eggs prepared in the same old way.)

TOMATO OMELET

½ onion
1 garlic clove
3 tablespoons butter

2 eggs
1 tomato
1 cup sprouts

Chop onion and crush garlic. Sauté together in butter. Beat eggs well. Chop tomato. Add all ingredients together and cover. Cook until set. (Another method: pour beaten eggs into separate pan; cook slowly until set. Add ingredients, fold eggs over once and cook until desired degree of doneness.)

EGGS FOO YUNG

¼ cup onion	2 tablespoons soy oil
1½ cups sprouts	4 eggs
1½ cups mushrooms	1 tablespoon tamari or soy sauce

Mince vegetables. Sauté in oil. Beat eggs well. Add sautéed vegetables to eggs and tamari, mixing thoroughly. Spoon mixture into hot oil and brown slowly. (This is a crunchy and delightful way to prepare eggs that don't taste like eggs).

AV-EGG-CADO

3 eggs	3 ripe avocados

Hard-boil eggs and mince. Halve avocados, removing seed. Spoon out avocado meat, mash and mix with eggs. Replace mixture in shell. Chill.

MERINGUE KISSES

This and the following recipe are simple, healthful cookies, good enough for company.

2 egg whites	1 cup chopped nuts or grated
1 cup maple sugar or raw sugar	coconut

Preheat oven to 250° F. Beat egg whites until stiff and dry. Slowly add sugar and nuts or coconut. Bake for 1 hour or until dry.

DATE MACAROONS

2 egg whites   1 cup chopped dates
1 cup powdered date sugar

Preheat oven to 325° F. Beat egg whites until stiff and dry. Fold in powdered sugar and chopped dates. (Powder date sugar in blender.) Drop by spoonful on well-oiled cookie sheet. Bake for 30 minutes until lightly browned.

EGG NUT SQUARES

This healthful, high-protein dessert is great if you are trying to avoid grains.

3 eggs   ⅓ cup honey
¼ teaspoon salt   1 cup ground nuts

Preheat oven to 350° F. Separate eggs. Beat yolks with salt and honey until thick and well-mixed. Beat whites until stiff, then fold in nuts and yolk mixture. Turn into a buttered 8″ x 8″ pan and bake for 30 minutes. Cool before cutting into squares.

CHEESE

SWEET PEPPER AND CHEESE

This unusual spread contains no mayonnaise.

1 sweet red pepper   2 cups grated natural cheese
½ cup pure wine or grape
  vinegar

Chop pepper finely. Marinate 24 hours in vinegar. Simmer

5 to 10 minutes until pepper is tender. Mix with grated cheese. Spread on green pepper segments or whole grain bread.

CHEESE BALLS

1 cup sharp natural cheese	*½ cup rice oil*
2 cups rice flour	*¼ teaspoon chopped chili pepper*

Preheat oven to 400° F. Grate cheese. Combine all ingredients. Chill well, then roll into small balls. Bake on lightly greased cookie sheet for 10 minutes.

CHEESE SAUCE

1 cup milk	*2 tablespoons starch or flour*
2 tablespoons butter	*¾ cup grated natural cheese*

Heat milk, but do not boil. Melt butter and add flour or starch. Stirring constantly, slowly add hot milk until mixture thickens. Stir in grated cheese and continue stirring until it is completely melted.

MILK

COTTAGE CHEESE

This is a cumbersome, messy and old recipe, but it's the only way to experience the way great-grandmother did it. The result is superior to the commercial variety.

Place ½ gallon milk in a covered jar and place in a warm (not hot) location. Allow milk to sour until whey and curd are separated. Drain the curd through cheese cloth until it is firm. Cool for a few hours, then beat until it achieves the consistency of cottage cheese you prefer.

POTATO SOUP

3 cups milk
2 cups diced potatoes

½ cup diced onion
2 teaspoons butter

Heat milk and add all ingredients. Simmer (do not boil) until potatoes are tender.

YOGURT DIP

Some people find that, although they cannot tolerate milk or most milk products, they can handle yogurt. It is an ancient food, a diet staple of certain middle European countries whose people are noted for longevity. It is rich in acidophilus. The Russians frequently feed fermented milk to infants, who rarely display milk allergies.

1 cup plain yogurt
¼ cup chopped pickles

1 tablespoon pickle juice

Combine all ingredients, mix well and chill. Use as a salad dressing or as a dip for raw vegetables.

YOGURT SOUP

⅓ cup raisins
⅓ cup milk
3 cups plain yogurt
½ onion

⅓ cup cucumber
6 ice cubes
Dill weed

Cover raisins with cold water and let stand until they are plump, about 30 minutes. Pour milk, yogurt, onion, raisins and cucumber into blender with 6 ice cubes. Blend thoroughly. Cover and chill until ready to serve. Garnish with dill weed.

YOGURT DRESSING

Combine 1 cup of plain yogurt with ⅓ cup of fresh fruit juice. Good as a fruit salad dressing or as a vegetable dip.

HONEY ICE CREAM

6 eggs   *1¾ cups honey*
½ gallon milk or cream

Separate eggs. Combine milk and honey. Heat slightly, then chill. Beat egg whites until stiff, yolks until thick. Fold into milk and honey mixture. Fill ice cream freezer can ⅔ full of mixture, adding milk if necessary, and freeze.

CHOCOLATE ICE CREAM

½ gallon milk or cream   *⅓ cup cocoa or carob powder*
8 ounces maple syrup

Pour 3 cups milk and syrup into blender. Blend at low speed, adding cocoa or carob. When well blended, pour into ice cream freezer can, adding remaining milk. Freeze.

STRAWBERRY ICE CREAM

6 cups strawberries   *1½ cups honey*
4 to 6 cups milk   *2 teaspoons kelp (optional)*
1 cup powdered milk

Hull strawberries. Combine all ingredients in ice cream freezer, adding milk to fill can ¾ full. Freeze. (Kelp will stabilize the mixture).

Note: Ice cream made in refrigerator/freezer trays is not very good—hard and unpalatable.

PEACH ICE CREAM

4 pounds fresh peaches   1 quart milk or cream
¾ cup honey

Pit and mash peaches. Add honey and milk, combine well and freeze in ice cream freezer.

RICE

BASIC RICE

This is a traditional Chinese method of preparation.

1 cup brown rice   2¼ cups cold water

Rinse rice well. Drain. Add cold water and bring to a boil over high heat. Boil 2 to 3 minutes, until crater-like holes appear on surface. Cover pan tightly, reduce heat and cook 50 minutes. Remove pan from heat, but do not uncover. Let it rest for 10 minutes. Remove cover and fluff.

FLUFFY RICE

¼ cup rice bran oil   2¼ cups water
1 cup brown rice

Heat oil and add rice, stirring until the rice is brown. Add water and cover. Simmer for 50 minutes. (In tropical countries, the rice is customarily browned in oil first to separate the grains, then steamed.)

FRIED RICE

You can vary color and flavor by using other vegetables

instead of, or in addition to, the pepper. Try small pieces of tomato, onion, chives, parsley or celery.

3 tablespoons rice oil   *1 cup cooked rice*
¼ cup green pepper

Heat oil in skillet. Combine pepper and rice and add to skillet. Turn frequently as rice browns.

SESAME RICE

1 cup rice   *2 cups water*
¼ cup rice oil   *2 tablespoons tamari or soy sauce*
3 tablespoons sesame seed

Brown rice in oil. Toast sesame seeds and add to rice. Add water. Simmer 50 minutes. Fluff with tamari and serve.

RICE CASSEROLE

1 green pepper   *2 tomatoes*
1 banana pepper   *2 cups water*
½ cup rice bran oil   *pinch chili powder*
1 cup brown rice

Chop peppers. Heat oil and stir in peppers and rice. Brown. Add tomatoes, water and chili powder. Cover and simmer for 50 minutes.

RICE NUT BREAD

4 eggs   *½ cup rice oil*
4 ounces ground nuts   *2 tablespoons honey*
½ pound rice flour

Preheat oven to 350° F. Beat eggs. Mix together with all other ingredients. Bake in greased loaf pan for 45 minutes.

BANANA RICE BREAD

This is particularly good for breakfast—a tasty, wheatless bread.

¼ cup rice oil	1½ cups rice flour
¾ cup raw sugar	2 teaspoons baking powder
1 cup mashed bananas	½ teaspoon soda

Preheat oven to 325° F. Combine oil and sugar. Add other ingredients and mix well. Bake in greased loaf pan for 40 minutes.

RICE PANCAKES

1 cup rice polish	¼ cup maple sugar
5 tablespoons rice oil	¼ teaspoon soda

Mix ingredients, adding enough water to obtain desired consistency. The thinner the batter, the crisper the pancakes. Bake on hot greased griddle, turning once. Serve with maple syrup.

RICE CRUST

This is a crunchy snack whether sprinkled with cinnamon, used as a pizza crust, cobbler topping or pie crust.

¼ cup rice oil	⅓ cup water
¾ cup rice flour	

Preheat oven to 425° F. Work oil into flour. Add enough water to make soft dough. Press dough as thinly as possible into oiled pan. Bake for 12 minutes or until brown.

RICE PUDDING

4 cups milk	¼ cup honey
2 cups rice	

Preheat oven to 225° F. Combine milk, rice and honey. Bake for 3 hours, stirring every 30 minutes. Cool, then chill. (Can also be served warm.)

RICE SPICE CAKE

2½ cups rice flour	½ cup rice oil
⅛ teaspoon ground cloves	2 eggs
1¼ teaspoons cinnamon	1½ cups applesauce (or mashed
½ teaspoon nutmeg	bananas)
3 teaspoons baking powder	3 tablespoons sour cream

Preheat oven to 375° F. Sift dry ingredients together. Blend oil, eggs, fruit sauce and sour cream. Mix all ingredients together thoroughly. Bake in a greased 8″ × 13″ pan for 30 minutes.

RICE SPONGE CAKE

4 eggs	½ cup maple sugar or raw sugar
½ cup rice flour	

Preheat oven to 300° F. Separate eggs. Whip whites until stiff, gradually adding sugar. Beat yolks until light. Add sifted flour to yolks, then fold batter slowly into whites. Bake in tube pan for 20 minutes or until done.

RICE-CAROB BROWNIES

½ cup rice oil	⅔ cup honey
⅓ cup carob powder	¾ cup rice flour
2 eggs	1 teaspoon baking powder

Preheat oven to 350° F. Heat oil, blend in carob powder and cool. Beat eggs until blended and continue to beat while adding honey. Add flour, baking powder and carob mixture. Mix well and spread in well-greased 8″ × 8″ baking pan. Let stand 30 minutes, then bake for 30 minutes.

APRI-RICE BARS

½ cup rice oil
2 eggs
¾ cup honey
1½ cups rice flour

3 teaspoons baking powder
½ teaspoon cinnamon
½ teaspoon nutmeg
1 cup stewed apricots

Preheat oven to 400° F. Beat oil, eggs and ½ cup honey. Stir in dry ingredients. Spread half of mixture in bottom of 9″ × 9″ baking pan. Chop apricots and mix with remaining honey. Layer over mixture in pan bottom, then top with remaining batter. Bake for 30 minutes. Cool and cut into bars.

HONEY SPICE RICE COOKIES

1½ cups honey
1 cup rice oil
3¾ cups rice flour
4¼ teaspoons baking powder

¼ teaspoon soda
1 teaspoon cinnamon
1 teaspoon ground cloves
1 teaspoon allspice

Preheat oven to 350° F. Heat honey and oil for about a minute. Cool. Sift dry ingredients and add to honey mixture. Mix well. Roll thin and cut with cookie cutter or into rounds, using a drinking glass. Bake for 12 to 15 minutes.

RICE WAFERS

¼ cup maple sugar or raw sugar
¼ cup butter
½ cup rice flour

1 tablespoon grated lemon rind
1 egg

Preheat oven to 350° F. Cream sugar into butter. Mix other ingredients and blend into butter. Roll thin and cut. Bake for 5 to 7 minutes.

RYE

RYE FLAKES

6 cups water   2 cups rye flakes
2 tablespoons oil

Boil water. Heat oil in another pan. Sauté flakes in oil, about 5 minutes. Add boiling water. Cover well and simmer 20 minutes, stirring occasionally.

RYE BERRY CASSEROLE

1 cup rye berries   ½ purple cabbage
1½ cups water   ½ teaspoon salt (optional)
1 onion

Preheat oven to 350° F. Simmer rye berries in water 1½ hours or until tender. Dice onion and shred cabbage. Steam vegetables and add to rye. Bake in oiled casserole for 15 minutes.

RYE BREAD

This recipe has no wheat or gluten flour, so it makes a very heavy bread.

1½ tablespoons yeast   ¼ cup molasses
1¼ cups lukewarm water   2 teaspoons salt
3 tablespoons oil   4 cups rye flour

Preheat oven to 425° F. Dissolve yeast in ½ cup warm water.

Mix remaining water with oil and molasses. Mix salt and flour. Add half the flour, stirring until smooth. Knead in remaining flour for 15 minutes. Let rise until doubled in bulk (about 1 hour). Beat down, knead another 100 times. Shape into 2 small loaves in well-greased pans. Let rise until double in bulk, about 45 minutes. Bake for 10 minutes, then reduce heat to 350° F. and bake for an additional 30 minutes.

SCOTCH SHORTBREAD

1 cup butter
¾ cup natural brown sugar

2¼ cups rye flour
¼ teaspoon salt (optional)

Preheat oven to 375° F. Cream butter and sugar. Mix in flour and salt. Shape into rolls (about 1½" diameter) and refrigerate 4 hours. Cut into ⅛" slices and bake on greased cookie sheet for 10 minutes.

RYE ZUCCHINI BREAD

This is an especially good use for rye flour. The resulting bread is good for breakfast, dinner or sweet cream sandwiches.

1 cup oil
2 eggs
1¾ cups honey
2 cups grated zucchini
3 cups rye flour

1 teaspoon salt
1 teaspoon soda
1 teaspoon baking powder
3 teaspoons cinnamon

Preheat oven to 325° F. Beat eggs. Add oil, honey and zucchini. Sift dry ingredients and add to zucchini mixture. Bake in two oiled loaf pans for 1 hour.

GINGERYEBREAD

½ cup butter or oil
1 egg
1 cup molasses
1 cup water
2½ cups rye flour

½ teaspoon salt
1 teaspoon ginger
1 teaspoon cinnamon
1 teaspoon soda

Preheat oven to 350° F. Cream butter. Beat in egg and add molasses. Mix well. Heat water and add alternately with sifted dry ingredients. Mix thoroughly and pour into greased 9″ × 13″ pan. Bake for 40 minutes.

CHOCOLATE CHIP COOKIES

⅓ cup oil
6 tablespoons raw sugar
6 tablespoons raw brown sugar
1 egg

1¼ cups rye flour
½ teaspoon soda
½ teaspoon salt
1 cup carob chips

Preheat oven to 375° F. Cream oil, sugar and egg. Mix in dry ingredients. Add carob. Drop by spoonfuls on greased cookie sheet and bake for 10 to 12 minutes.

MOLASSES BARS

1¾ cups rye flour
½ cup oil
1 teaspoon cinnamon

¾ cup molasses
1 egg
1½ teaspoons baking powder

Preheat oven to 350° F. Mix all ingredients together. Bake in 9″ × 13″ pan for 25 minutes. Allow to cool and cut into serving bars.

RYE CRACKERS

1¾ cups rye flour
2 tablespoons oil

¼ teaspoon salt
4 tablespoons water

Preheat oven to 325° F. Mix flour, oil and salt by hand. Add water. Knead. Roll out and cut into rounds. Bake on oiled sheet for 12 minutes.

RYE GINGERSNAPS

½ cup oil	2¼ cups rye flour
1 cup brown sugar	2 teaspoons soda
1 egg	1 teaspoon cinnamon
¼ cup molasses	1 teaspoon ginger

Preheat oven to 375° F. Mix oil, brown sugar, egg and molasses. Beat in dry ingredients. Cover and chill 1 hour. Drop by teaspoonfuls onto greased baking sheet. Sprinkle with sugar and bake for 10 to 12 minutes.

OATS

OATMEAL BREAD WITH YEAST

This is a crunchy, heavy bread. It is dry and somewhat mealy.

1½ tablespoons yeast	2 tablespoons oil
1¼ cups warm water	1 cup rolled oats
3 tablespoons honey	2½ cups oat flour
salt	½ cup raisins

Preheat oven to 375° F. Dissolve yeast in water and let stand 10 minutes. Stir in honey, salt and oil. Beat in oats and half the flour. Add remaining flour and raisins. Cover and let rise until doubled in bulk. Stir hard for 1 minute. Place in greased loaf pan, let rise again. Bake for 35-45 minutes.

OATMEAL BREAD (NO YEAST)

This is a first-rate breakfast bread, with just the right amount of sweetness.

1½ cups boiling water
1 cup oats
½ cup butter
2 cups brown sugar
1⅓ cups oat flour

2 eggs
1 tablespoon cinnamon
1 teaspoon soda
1 cup raisins
1 cup nuts

Preheat oven to 350° F. Pour water over oats and let stand for 20 minutes. Cream butter and sugar. Mix remaining ingredients into butter. Bake in greased 9″ × 13″ pan for 40 minutes.

DATE-OAT TORTE

This is a good lunchbox addition and fine for breakfast or snacktime. You can substitute other fresh or dried fruits for the dates.

1½ cups dates
¾ cup date sugar
1 cup water

2 cups oats
½ teaspoon soda
½ cup butter

Preheat oven to 350° F. Pit and chop dates. Mix with ¼ cup sugar and ½ cup water. Simmer until thick. Mix in remaining ingredients. Spread half of dough in 8″ × 8″ greased pan. Cover with fruit. Top with remaining dough. Bake for 30 minutes.

OATMEAL CEREAL

Try this recipe with steel-cut oats. It has a totally different consistency and a somewhat different taste. You can also cook it with dried fruit for a sweet accent.

½ cup steel-cut or rolled oats   2 cups water

Combine in saucepan and cover. Simmer over low heat for 20 to 30 minutes.

GRANOLA

This is more economical than buying the ready-mixed versions, and *you* get to pick the ingredients and the proportions. Check to see that foods you include are from the same food families.

2 cups rolled oats	1 cup chopped almonds
1/3 cup maple syrup or honey	1 cup dried apricots, diced

Preheat oven to 325° F. Mix all ingredients together. Spread thinly on a cookie sheet and bake for 20 minutes or until light brown.

OATEN SESAME

When you want something sweet and crunchy, try these cookies.

1 cup sesame seeds	1 cup rolled oats
1 cup tahini (sesame butter)	1 cup maple syrup

Preheat oven to 375° F. Toast seeds. Combine with tahini, oats and syrup. Mix well. Drop by spoonfuls on greased cookie sheet and bake for 20 minutes.

APPLE OAT CRISPS

2 cups apples	1/3 cup brown sugar
1 teaspoon cinnamon	1/4 cup oil
1 1/2 cups rolled oats	1/2 teaspoon soda

Preheat oven to 350° F. Slice apples. Arrange in greased baking dish. Sprinkle with cinnamon. Combine remaining ingredients and spread over apple slices. Bake for 40 minutes.

OATMEAL COOKIES

2½ cups oat flour
1½ cups brown sugar
1 cup butter
1 teaspoon soda

½ cup warm water
2½ cups oats
2 teaspoons poppy seeds
(optional)

Preheat oven to 350° F. Sift flour and sugar together. Add butter. Mix soda with warm water and stir into oats. Add all other ingredients, mix well and chill until firm. Roll out to ¼" thickness and cut into rounds. Bake for 10 minutes.

OAT AND NUT CRUNCH

⅓ cup butter
⅓ cup raw sugar
2 tablespoons water
1 cup oats

⅓ cup brown sugar
½ teaspoon baking powder
1 cup chopped nuts

Preheat oven to 350° F. Cream butter and sugar. Beat in water, then dry ingredients. Drop from teaspoon onto greased cookie sheet. Bake for 10 minutes.

PEANUT BUTTER COOKIES

¼ cup brown sugar
2 tablespoons peanut butter
2 teaspoons peanut oil
¼ cup water

1½ cups oat flour
2 teaspoons baking powder
½ cup chopped peanuts

Preheat oven to 400° F. Cream sugar, peanut butter and oil. Add water, then dry ingredients. Stir in peanuts. Drop by teaspoonfuls onto greased cookie sheet. Press each cookie with fork tines. Bake until golden brown.

WHEAT

YEASTLESS DINNER ROLLS

½ cup oil
¼ cup sugar
1 egg
¼ cup milk or water

2 cups whole wheat flour
½ teaspoon salt
3½ teaspoons baking powder

Preheat oven to 375° F. Combine oil, sugar, egg and liquid. Knead in flour, salt and baking powder. Shape into rolls and bake for 15 minutes.

CROUTONS

Garlic, onions or leeks
2 tablespoons butter

Whole wheat bread

Chop seasoning(s) and combine with butter. Spread on bread. Cut bread into sticks or cubes and broil until brown. Another method: Dry out in slow oven (200° F.) for 2 hours.

THREE-IN-ONE DOUGH

2 tablespoons yeast
1 cup warm water
1 cup hot water
¾ cup oil

½ cup honey
2 teaspoons salt
2 eggs
6½ cups whole wheat flour

Preheat oven. Dissolve yeast in warm water. In another bowl, mix hot water, oil, honey and salt. Add eggs, diluted yeast, then flour. Yield: 3 dozen rolls.
DINNER ROLLS: Shape into rolls. Allow to rise. Bake at 425° F. for 12 minutes.
CINNAMON ROLLS: Roll into thin rectangle and spread with butter and honey. Sprinkle with raisins, nuts and/or cinnamon.

roll up dough and slice. Bake at 400° F. for 15 minutes.
HAMBURGER BUNS: Roll dough ½" thick. Cut out rounds
with custard cup. Place on greased sheet. Allow to rise,
then bake at 400° F. for 12 minutes.

DOUGH-NOTS

When you want your own home-made, whole wheat, non-commercial doughnut, try this. . .but don't expect the lightness
of the great American "dunker." These don't rise as much,
so they're much heavier.

2 eggs
1 cup raw sugar
1 cup milk
5 tablespoons oil
½ teaspoon salt

1 teaspoon ground or grated
  lemon rind
4 cups whole wheat flour
4 teaspoons baking powder
½ teaspoon cinnamon

Beat eggs. Add sugar, milk and oil. Beat dry ingredients
together and add to egg mixture. Mix well, cut into doughnut
shapes (use rim of large glass for the doughnut, shot glass
rim for the hole) and fry.

SHOO FLY PIE

LIQUID MIXTURE:

½ cup molasses
½ teaspoon baking soda

½ cup hot water

CRUMB MIXTURE:

1½ cups flour
¼ teaspoon salt
1 cup raw brown sugar

1 teaspoon cinnamon
¼ cup oil

Preheat oven to 450° F. Combine dry ingredients. Work in oil to create crumbs. Using unbaked pie shell, start with a layer of crumbs, then alternate with layers of liquid mixture, ending with a crumb layer on top. Bake for 15 minutes, then reduce heat to 350° F. and bake an additional 20 minutes.

CARROT BREAD

²/₃ cup peanut oil
³/₄ cup honey
2 eggs
1½ cups whole wheat flour
1 teaspoon cinnamon

2 teaspoons nutmeg
½ teaspoon salt
1 teaspoon baking powder
1 cup chopped peanuts
1½ cups grated carrots

Preheat oven to 350° F. Cream oil and honey. Add eggs, then dry ingredients which have been sifted together. Add carrot shreds and peanuts. Mix thoroughly. Pour into greased loaf pan and bake for 1 hour.

APRICOT TEA LOAF

³/₄ cup dried apricots
1 cup water
2 cups whole wheat flour
3 teaspoons baking powder
1 teaspoon salt

1 cup raw sugar
3 tablespoons oil or melted butter
1 egg
½ cup orange juice

Preheat oven to 350° F. Wash apricots and cover with ½ cup boiling water. Let stand overnight. Drain and save ¼ cup juice. Chop apricots fine and add ¼ cup juice. Combine flour, baking powder and salt, and add to apricot mixture. Cream sugar and oil, and add egg, orange juice, ½ cup water and apricot mixture. Mix well. Bake for 1½ hours.

EGGLESS COFFEE CAKE

3 cups whole wheat flour
½ teaspoon salt
2 teaspoons cinnamon
½ cup oil

2 teaspoons soda
1 cup cream or buttermilk
1 cup honey

Preheat oven to 350° F. Sift flour, salt and cinnamon together and crumble by working in oil. Reserve ½ cup for topping. Dissolve soda in cream, add honey and mix with crumbs. Pour into greased and floured 9″ × 13″ pan. Add topping. Bake for 30 minutes.

APPLE CAKE

3 cups fresh apple
2 eggs
1½ cups oil
½ teaspoon soda

1 cup honey
3 cups whole wheat flour
½ teaspoon cinnamon
½ teaspoon salt

Preheat oven to 350° F. Chop apples. Beat eggs. Mix all ingredients together. Place in tube pan and bake for 1½ hours.

BROWNIE CUPCAKES

4 squares semi-sweet chocolate
1 cup butter
1 cup flour

1¾ cups raw sugar
4 eggs, plus water to make 1 cup

Preheat oven to 325° F. Melt chocolate and butter. Combine with all other ingredients. Bake in greased muffin tins for 35 minutes.

HONEY BROWNIES

Hint: when using carob powder, melt or heat it in oil or water. It will taste more like chocolate.

BROWNIES:

½ cup oil
6 ounces carob or chocolate
   chips
2 eggs, beaten

2 tablespoons honey
½ cup flour
½ teaspoon baking powder
¼ teaspoon salt

ICING:

6 tablespoons raw sugar

2 tablespoons honey

Preheat oven to 350° F. Melt oil and carob over warm water. Cool. Beat in eggs and honey. Sift dry ingredients together and add to egg mixture. Spread in 8″×8″ greased pan. Bake for 30 minutes.
ICING: Powder sugar in blender. Mix with honey and spread on brownies while warm.

BARLEY

BARLEY CASSEROLE

1 cup barley
1 cup boiling water
1 butternut squash

2 yellow squash
1 white squash

Add barley to water and simmer for 20 minutes. Peel butternut squash. Chop all varieties of squash and add to barley. Add water as necessary. Simmer about 30 minutes or until done.

BARLEY SOUP

This is a hearty winter dish.

2 onions
½ pound mushrooms
2 tablespoons soy oil
1 cup barley or millet

4 cups water
2 teaspoons salt
2 tablespoons tamari or soy sauce

Peel and chop onions. Clean and slice mushrooms. Heat oil and sauté onions and barley for 5 minutes. Add water and simmer slowly for 1 hour. Add mushrooms, salt and tamari. Simmer for an additional 5 minutes and serve.

BARLEY BREAD

1¾ cups barley flour
4½ teaspoons baking powder
½ teaspoon salt

1¼ teaspoons oil
½ cup water
2 tablespoons honey

Preheat oven to 375° F. Sift dry ingredients and add oil. Combine water and honey and add to flour mixture. Bake in small loaf pan for 25 minutes.

BARLEY CHIFFON CAKE

5 egg yolks
1¼ cups raw sugar
¾ cup orange juice
3 tablespoons grated orange rind

1¾ cups barley flour
4 teaspoons baking powder
7 egg whites
½ cup oil

Preheat oven to 350° F. Beat egg yolks until thick. Mix sugar, oil or orange juice and rind into yolks. Sift dry ingredients and add to batter. Beat egg whites until stiff. Fold batter by hand into egg whites. Bake in tube pan for 1 hour.

BUCKWHEAT

Buckwheat is not a grain; therefore, you'll find it decidedly different from other flours. Generally, what is served as buckwheat is buckwheat mixed with wheat. An all-buckwheat recipe will taste unfamiliar. You're adventurous, aren't you?

BUCKWHEAT CEREAL

½ cup buckwheat   *1 cup water*

Combine and simmer 30 minutes or until tender.

RAISED BUCKWHEAT CAKES

2 cups milk or water   *1 tablespoon molasses*
1 teaspoon yeast   *1 teaspoon soda*
1¾ cups buckwheat flour   *¼ cup oil*
½ teaspoon salt

Scald the milk and let it cool. Stir in yeast. Add buckwheat and salt, stirring until mixture is smooth. Cover and let rise for 12 hours. Stir in molasses. Dissolve soda in ¼ cup of water and add. Stir in oil. Bake cakes on well greased, hot griddle, turning once.

BUCKWHEAT PANCAKES

2 tablespoons oil   *½ teaspoon salt*
3¼ cups sour milk   *1 teaspoon soda*
2 teaspoons molasses   *1½ cups buckwheat flour*
½ teaspoon baking powder

Combine oil, milk and molasses. Sift dry ingredients and stir into mixture, blending well. Drop on hot, greased griddle and cook until done, turning once.

MINIMAL INGREDIENT BUCKWHEAT CAKES

¾ cup water   *2 teaspoons molasses (optional)*
½ cup buckwheat flour   *½ teaspoon salt (optional)*

Mix ingredients until batter is full of bubbles. Fry on a hot, oiled griddle.

ARROWROOT

Arrowroot is like a grain, but it's not a grain. It is a tropical plant with tuberous roots and an excellent thickener that can be used in place of cornstarch.

ARROWROOT BATTER

1 cup seeds or nuts	*½ cup arrowroot starch*
1 cup water	*1½ tablespoons oil*
2 teaspoons baking powder	*2 tablespoons honey*

Puree seeds or nuts with water in blender. Mix well with remaining ingredients.
TO MAKE A COBBLER: Pour batter over prepared fruit and bake at 350° F. for 35 minutes.
FOR PANCAKES: Drop batter on hot, oiled griddle.

NUT BALLS

½ cup raw brown sugar	*4 tablespoons oil*
1 cup arrowroot flour	*7 tablespoons cold water*
¼ teaspoon salt	*3 tablespoons chopped nuts*
2 teaspoons baking powder	

Preheat oven to 375° F. Mix dry ingredients and work oil into mixture. Add water and stir until smooth. Add nuts. Shape batter into small balls. Bake for 15 minutes.

DATE ARROWROOT LOAF

½ pound dates   *1 cup arrowroot flour*
4 eggs   *2 cups date sugar*
1½ teaspoons baking powder   *4 cups chopped walnuts*

Preheat oven to 300° F. Pit and chop dates. Beat eggs. Sift
dry ingredients together, adding eggs. Stir in dates and nuts
until they are thoroughly coated. Pack into three small, well-
greased loaf pans. Bake for 1 hour. Remove from pan while
warm.

POTATO STARCH

(Another excellent grain substitute)

POTATO SPONGE CAKE

6 eggs   *2 teaspoons baking powder*
1 cup raw sugar   *3 tablespoons water*
1 cup potato starch *1 teaspoon lemon juice*

Preheat oven to 300° F. Separate eggs. Beat yolks well,
gradually adding sugar. Mix dry ingredients and add to yolks.
Add water and lemon juice. Beat egg whites until stiff and
fold into batter. Pour into tube pan and bake for 1 hour.

POTATO FRITTERS

½ cup potato starch   *½ cup milk*
½ cup rice flour   *1 egg, beaten*
1½ teaspoons baking powder   *1 tablespoon honey*
¼ teaspoon salt

Sift dry ingredients and add milk. Stir in egg and honey

until batter is smooth. Drop by spoonfuls into hot oil. Cook until golden brown.

SPUD WAFFLES

If you're allergic to wheat, you can still enjoy waffles. Here's a favorite wheat substitute.

⅓ cup potato starch
2 teaspoons baking powder
⅔ cup soy flour
¼ teaspoon salt

1⅛ cups milk
3 tablespoons soy oil
2 teaspoons honey

Sift dry ingredients. Combine with milk. Gradually stir in oil mixed with honey. Stir until smooth. Bake in heated waffle iron.

NUTS AND SEEDS

The following recipes for candies and cookies are healthful and nutritious—a way to divert the youngsters (and some oldsters, too) from refined sugar confections. Try these when you want something that includes protein and minerals. . . and still tastes like a treat.

SESAME SEED CANDY

2 cups sesame seeds
1 cup honey

2 tablespoons water

Preheat oven to 425° F. Spread seeds in bottom of 8″ × 12″ pan. Dribble honey over seeds. Pour in water and mix together. Bake until seeds begin to brown. Harden in freezer before cutting.

PEANUT BRITTLE

2 cups raw sugar
2 cups peanuts

1 teaspoon salt
2 teaspoons baking soda
(optional)

Melt sugar, stirring frequently until light brown in color. Pour over nuts tossed with salt and soda in oiled pan. Cool thoroughly.

PEANUT BUTTER MERINGUES

2 egg whites
3/4 cup raw sugar

1/2 cup peanut butter
1/4 teaspoon salt

Preheat oven to 325° F. Whip egg whites until stiff, gradually adding sugar and salt. In separate bowl, beat peanut butter until soft. Fold peanut butter into egg whites. Drop on greased cookie sheet and bake for 20 minutes or until lightly browned.

CAROB CANDY

1/4 cup honey
1/2 cup carob powder

1/2 cup peanut butter or tahini
1/2 cup peanuts or sesame seeds

Mix honey, carob and nut butter. Shape into balls and roll in ground nuts or seeds. Chill well.

TOASTED NUTS

Almonds or cashews

Tamari or soy sauce

Preheat oven to 250° F. Toss nuts with enough tamari to coat well. Brown nuts for several hours until toasty and crisp.

TOFFEE

2 cups butter
2½ cups raw turbinado sugar
¼ cup water

1 cup chopped nuts
1 package carob or chocolate
  chips

Combine butter, sugar, water and ½ cup nuts. Cook to hard crack stage. Pour on greased cookie sheet. Refrigerate until crackly. Melt chips and spread over candy. Sprinkle with ground nuts and let harden. Turn over and spread on other side. Chill.

ALMOND COOKIES

3 cups ground almonds
3 tablespoons honey
1½ tablespoons almond oil

1 tablespoon lemon juice
1 teaspoon lemon rind, grated
½ teaspoon cinnamon

Preheat oven to 250° F. Combine ingredients and sparingly add boiling water to make a stiff dough. Roll out dough as thinly as possible on oiled cookie sheet, using a wet rolling pin. Cut in squares. Bake for 25 minutes. Cool.

PECAN PIE

CRUST:

3 cups ground pecans

⅓ cup butter

FILLING:

1½ cups molasses
4 eggs
2 tablespoons flour or carob
  powder

1¼ cups pecans
1 tablespoon butter

Preheat oven to 300° F. Lightly brown pecans in butter. Press into buttered pie pan. Bake for 10 minutes.

Preheat oven to 350° F. Mix all ingredients together well. Pour into crust. Bake for 40 minutes.

PHYSIOLOGICAL AND PSYCHOLOGICAL SYMPTOMS OF ALLERGY

MUSCLES: Tightness; stiffness; aching, especially tension in neck, back and lower extremities.

JOINTS: Swelling, redness, stiffness, aching, sensation of warmth.

LUNGS: Coughing, sneezing, reduced air flow, retraction, feeling of heaviness or tightness, hyperventilation, shallow or rapid breathing.

HEART: Rapid or slowed pulse or heartbeat, violent or throbbing pulse, chest pain.

GENITOURINARY SYSTEM: Frequent urination or urge to void, feeling of urgency or pressure, painful or difficult urination, genital itch.

GASTROINTESTINAL SYSTEM, ABDOMEN: Belching, nausea, vomiting; full, bloated feeling; pain, cramps; flatus, gas rumbling; diarrhea, constipation; excessive or lack of hunger or thirst; hyperacidity; gall bladder symptoms.

SKIN: Local or general itching; moist skin, sweating; flushing, hives; rashes; pallor, white or gray tones, bruising.

THROAT, LARYNX AND SPEECH: Itching, sore, tight, swollen throat; difficulty in swallowing, choking; excessive salivation and/or mucous; bad metallic taste; hoarseness, tic or fuzzy speech; stuttering or stammering; inability to express what one wishes; inability to control word sequence, or reversal of words; wishing to say one thing and saying another; slow and difficult coordination of speech.

FACE, NECK AND HEAD: Headache, migraine; tightness, pressure, throbbing or stabbing pain; burning, tingling sensation; tics, temporary paralysis; stiff neck; head retraction.

NOSE, SMELL: Sneezing, urge to sneeze; itching; discharge, stuffy feeling, obstruction; post-nasal drip, sinus discomfort; hypersensitivity to odors or inability to distinguish between odors.

EARS, HEARING: Itching; sensation of fullness or blocking; earache; reddening of ears; hearing louder or softer than reality; sensation of air rushing in ears; deafness; ringing, tinkling or buzzing sounds in ear; abnormal sensitivity to sound.

EYES, VISION: Ocular muscle incoordination or paralysis; inability to direct optic axes to same object; pupil changes; itching, burning, pain, heavy feeling; drooping upper eyelid; dark circles under eyes; tears; seeing larger or smaller than reality; blind spots; blurred vision; temporarily dimmed vision; double vision, sensitivity to light; inability to see in dark, visual hallucinations.

CENTRAL NERVOUS SYSTEM: Partial or total paralysis; epilepsy; convulsions; dizziness; lightheadedness, fainting; partial blackouts, unconsciousness; vertigo, sensation of imbalance; inability to read or understand words, jumbling of words; drowsiness, yawning attacks, extended deep sleep, insomnia, nightmares; fatigue, neurasthenia; lack of concentration, poor attention span, lowered mentality; unhappiness, sulkiness, depression, suicidal thoughts; agitation, excitability; talkativeness; unreasonable, erratic behavior; indecisive, irresponsible behavior; tense, anxious, restless, irritable behavior; explosive outbursts, hallucinations.

HOUSEHOLD CHEMICAL SUBSTITUTES

LAUNDRY AGENTS: For machine-washing clothes, rub
damp baking soda into dirty spots, then add ½ cup
baking soda to one medium washer-load of clothes. For
particularly dirty clothes, wash with regular detergent and
add ½ cup baking soda to rinse cycle, followed by
second rinse of clear water. Other products used with
success by some include Borax, Arm and Hammer washing powder, Amway's L.O.C. and Shakley's Basic H.

HOUSEHOLD CLEANSER: Dampen sink, toilet or bathtub.
Sprinkle with baking soda. Scrub with sponge. For particularly difficult jobs, clean with Borax and then baking
soda.

OVEN CLEANER: Sprinkle a small amount of water in oven,
then sprinkle ample amount of baking soda over oven.
Leave 30 minutes. Use steel wool pads and small amount
of water to loosen dirty area. Wipe clean with sponge.

BRASS AND COPPER POLISH: Dampen metal object. Apply
baking soda with sponge. Polish with soft cloth.

GLASS AND MIRROR CLEANER: Dampen cloth with vinegar and wipe off windows.

FABRIC FINISH SOFTENER: Fill basin with 3 parts water
to 1 part vinegar. Allow to soak overnight. Rinse vinegar
out of fabric.

FLOOR WAX: Choose wax that has a higher percentage of
the natural wax, carnauba, and less of the petroleum
products.

ROOM DEODORIZER: Partially fill bowls with baking soda
or vinegar and distribute about room.

REFRIGERATOR FRESHENER: Leave box of baking soda
open in refrigerator. Change boxes frequently.

STORING OR FREEZING FOOD: Store foods in glass or in bags made from cellophane, a wood fiber.

DISHES AND COOKWARE: Porcelain, glass and stainless steel do not volatize or transmit chemicals from themselves to the food within.

INSECTICIDE: Prepare ordinary mashed potatoes. To the potatoes, add ½ bottle of powdered boric acid. Stir thoroughly. Place spoonfuls on 2-inch squares of wax paper. Place balls in kitchen cupboards, under sink, in areas troubled by roaches and similar insects. Or mix boric acid, half and half, with sifted powdered sugar. Sprinkle in roach-infested areas.

CARPET PAD: Use mohair pads under area rugs or natural fiber carpet. Rubber or synthetic carpet pad is a major source of volatization, particularly when heated by sunlight or heat within the house. Carpeting may be found in wool or cotton. Oriental rugs are usually tolerable, especially older, antique rugs.

NONTOXIC REMEDIES

DEODORANT: Sprinkle soda on a damp wash cloth and apply to underarms.

TOOTHPASTE: Mix 1 part salt with 2 parts baking soda. Apply directly to toothbrush.

MOUTHWASH: Mix 1 teaspoon baking soda with a glass of water. Drink tea made from sage or birch leaves.

TOOTHACHE: Apply oil of cloves directly to tooth.

HICCOUGHS: Drink tea made from dill leaves.

SORE THROAT: Mix apple juice and honey. Heat and sip.

COLDS, NASAL CONGESTION: Mix apple juice and honey. Heat and sip. Drink tea made from catnip.

EARACHE: Heat 3 tablespoons of olive oil. Grind oregano into the oil. Apply directly to ear with cotton swab.

STOMACHACHE, INDIGESTION: Mix 1 teaspoon baking soda in glass of water. Drink, then follow with another glass of water. Or drink tea made from camomile or fennel.

DISINFECTANT: Apply garlic juice or a tea made from comfrey, goldenseal or marigold flowers around fresh wounds or cuts.

SUNBURN, SPRAINS, FROSTBITE: Apply witch hazel liberally.

FOOD RECIPE SUBSTITUTES

BUTTER: 1 cup equals $7/8$ cup oil (not recommended for cookies).

CHOCOLATE: 1 ounce chocolate is the equivalent of 3 tablespoons carob heated in $1\frac{1}{2}$ teaspoons oil.

COCONUT: Grate by grinding small chunks in blender. To make coconut meal, grind very finely and spread on foil to dry.

CORNSTARCH: Substitute whole wheat flour, rice flour, arrowroot starch or potato starch.

CREAM: 1 cup equals $\frac{3}{4}$ cup milk plus $\frac{1}{3}$ cup butter, mixed in blender.

EGG: 1 egg equals 1-$1\frac{1}{2}$ teaspoons of any of the following:
1. Soak $\frac{1}{2}$ pound apricots in 2 cups water overnight. Blend, strain and refrigerate.
2. To 3 cups cold water add 1 cup flax seed. Boil for 3 minutes, stirring constantly.

Or substitute 2 tablespoons water, 1 tablespoon oil and 2 tablespoons baking powder for 1 egg.

FLOUR: 1 cup of whole wheat flour is the equivalent of the following: $1\frac{1}{3}$ cups oats or oat flour, $1\frac{1}{4}$ cups rye flour, $\frac{3}{4}$ cup soy flour, $5/8$ cup potato starch, $\frac{1}{2}$ cup barley flour, $7/8$ cup rice flour, $\frac{3}{4}$ cup corn meal. Or substitute equal amounts of ground nuts or seeds. The easiest method is to cover the nuts or seeds with whatever liquid the recipe calls for and puree.

Thicken with arrowroot, barley, bean soup, buckwheat flour or flakes, nut or seed meal, poi, potato flour or starch, vegetables cooked and pureed.

MILK: Substitute an equal amount of any of the following:
1. Soya milk, made by gradually adding 1 quart soy flour to 4 cups water in blender. Strain. Heat drip-

pings for 15 minutes in double boiler, stirring frequently. Cool and refrigerate until needed.

2. Coconut milk, made by pureeing in blender ½ cup coconut or coconut meal in 1 cup water.

3. Nut or seed milk, made by pureeing in blender ½ cup nuts or seeds in 1 cup water.

SUGAR: 1 cup sugar is the equivalent of ⅔ cup honey; or 1 cup maple syrup; or ¾ cup molasses plus ¼ teaspoon baking soda.

SUGAR, POWDERED: Turn blender on. Slowly add turbinado sugar. Grind until powdery.

VANILLA: One-half teaspoon vanilla extract is the equivalent of 1 teaspoon ground vanilla bean. Or place vanilla bean in a quart jar of sugar. Use this vanilla sugar whenever vanilla is required in recipes.

COOKING HINTS

Cook whole grains such as wheat and rice in 3 parts water to 1 part grain. Cook with lid on.

Scramble eggs using a small amount of hot water in the skillet to prevent scorching.

Soak pinto beans at least an hour in water before cooking to reduce cooking time.

Sea salt may be added to any of the test foods.

When testing foods, cook a large amount so you won't be hungry before the next meal.

Unless a product is plainly labeled organic, it probably is not grown in any special way. This means it may contain contaminating residues of insecticides or chemical fertilizers.

The "juice" carrots one sometimes sees in health food stores are not necessarily organically grown.

Many of the candies and gums one sees in health food stores contain artificial sweeteners, flavors and colors.

Many imported foodstuffs may have been fumigated enroute to the U.S. This means they are possibly chemically contaminated.

Rye flour sold in the grocery store often has been mixed with wheat flour.

Not all "brown" flour is whole wheat. Color may have been added to make it look like whole wheat. Be sure the label says "stone ground."

Buckwheat is not a grain, but a member of the rhubarb family—it is helpful to those who are grain-sensitive.

Yeast contains corn and/or rye and/or barley. Red Star is the only corn-free brand. Yeast can be made by leaving out an uncovered mixture of potato flour, water, salt and sugar for several hours. Unfortunately, the quality of the resulting yeast varies greatly.

Most baking powders contain cornstarch, potato starch or tartaric acid, made from grapes.

Oils not distinctly labeled cold-pressed have been heated. This changes the molecular structure and may cause rancidity.

In recipes calling for water, use a more nutritious liquid whenever possible, such as milk, vegetable stock or fruit juice.

Nearly all cans are lined with plastic. Even canned goods in the health food stores, therefore, may contain aggravating substances if you are chemically sensitive.

Food stored in plastic bags should be aired 4 days if one is attempting to avoid chemical contamination.

Food may be safely wrapped in aluminum foil if the shiny surface of the foil is placed next to the food. The dull side is plastic-coated.

To increase the refrigerator life of fruits and vegetables, store in large glass jars with lids on. Most will keep for three weeks.

Freeze fruits in individual chunks on a cookie sheet before placing in cellophane bags for the freezer. Then, remove piece by piece, as needed.

Freezing fruit requires no syrup. Grapes, watermelon, cantaloupe, peaches, pears and cherries will all freeze with no preparation except washing.

How to Avoid Corn

METHODS OF EXPOSURE

Inhalation:
>   Fumes from cooking corn or corn products
>   Ironing starched clothes
>   Body powders and bath powders

Contact:
>   Starched clothing
>   Corn adhesives

Ingestion:
>   Corn and corn products
>   Glucose and dextrose sweeteners
>   Medications

FOODS THAT *MAY* CONTAIN CORN OR CORN PRODUCTS

adhesives
   envelopes, stamps,
   stickers, tapes
aspirin & other tablets
bacon
baking powder
beets, Harvard (canned)
beer
birth control pills
bourbon and other whiskies
brandy
bread and pastries
breath sprays and drops
cakes
candy
carbonated beverages
catsup
cereals, processed
cheese
chewing gum
chili, canned
chop suey, canned
chow mein, canned
coffee, instant
cola drinks
cookies
confectioner's sugar
corn flakes
cough syrup
cream pies
cream puffs

cups, paper
dates, confection
dentifrices
dextrose
egg nog, prepared
envelopes, sealing gum
fish, processed
flour, bleached
French dressing
fried foods, processed
Fritos
frostings, processed
fruits, canned and frozen
fruit juices, canned
fruit pies, processed
frying fats
gelatin capsules
gelatin dessert
glucose
graham crackers
grape juice, processed
gravies
grits
gums, chewing
gummed papers
   envelopes, labels
   stamps, tapes
gin
ginger ale
hair sprays
ham, cured and tenderized

ice cream
jam
Jell-o
jelly
laxatives
lemonade, processed
Life Savers
liquor
lollipops
lozenges, in excipients
margarine
meats, processed and cold cuts
ointments, in excipients
milk, in paper cartons
monosodium glutamate
paper containers
pastries
peanut butter
peas, canned
pickles
pies, creamed
plastic food wrappers
popcorn
pork and beans
powdered sugar
powders, face and body
puddings, processed
ravioli, canned
rice, processed

root beer
salt, seasoned
salad dressings, processed
sandwich spreads
sauces, processed
sausage
scotch
soft drinks
spaghetti
soups, processed
soy bean milk, processed
starch
suppositories, in excipients
syrups, processed
tablets, in excipients
talcum
tea, instant
toothpaste
tortillas
vanillin
vegetables, canned, creamed,
    frozen
vinegar, distilled
vitamins, in excipients
waffles, processed
weiners
whiskey
wine
yeast

FOODS THAT MAY CONTAIN MILK OR MILK PRODUCTS

au gratin foods, like potatoes or beans au gratin
baking powder biscuits
baker's bread
bavarian cream bisques
boiled salad dressings
bologna
butter
buttermilk
butter sauces
cakes
candies
cheese
chocolate or cocoa drinks
chowders
cookies
cream
creamed foods
cream sauces
cheeses
curd
custards
doughnuts
eggs, scrambled
escalloped dishes
gravy
hamburger buns
hash
hard sauces
hot cakes
ice cream

Junket
mashed potatoes
malted milk
meat loaf
milk chocolate
milk (condensed, dried, evaporated, fresh goat's, malted milk and powdered milk)
mixes for
  biscuits
  cakes
  cookies
  doughnuts
  muffins
  pancakes
  pie crust
  waffles and puddings
omelets
oleomargarine
quiche
rarebits
salad dressings
sherbets
soda crackers
soufflés
soups
whey
waffles
yogurt
zweibach

FOODS THAT MAY CONTAIN WHEAT

BEVERAGES: beer, bourbon, gin, malted milk, scotch and whiskey

BREADS: biscuits, crackers, muffins, popovers, pretzels, rolls and the following kinds of breads: corn, gluten, graham, pumpernickel, rye, soy and white bread

CEREALS: bran flakes, corn flakes, Cream of Wheat, crackers, Farina, Grapenuts, Krumbles, Muffets, Pep, Puffed Wheat, Ralston's Wheat Cereal, Rice Krispies, Shredded Wheat, Triscuits, Wheaties

FLOURS: buckwheat, corn, gluten, graham, lima bean, rice, rye, white and whole wheat

MISCELLANEOUS: bouillon cubes, chocolate candy, cooked mixed meat dishes, fats used for frying foods rolled in flour, fish rolled in flour, fowl rolled in flour, gravies, griddle cakes, hot cakes, ice cream cones, malt products or foods containing malt, meat rolled in flour, most cooked sausages (weiners, bologna, liverwurst lunch ham, hamburger, etc.), matzos, mayonnaise, pancake mixtures, sauces, synthetic pepper, some yeasts, thickening in ice creams, waffles, wheat cakes and wheat germ

PASTRIES AND DESSERTS: cakes, cookies, doughnuts, pies (including frozen), chocolate candy, candy bars and puddings

WHEAT PRODUCTS: bread and cracker crumbs, dumplings, hamburger mix, macaroni, noodles, rusk, spaghetti, vermicelli and zwieback

FOOD CONSTITUENTS OF
ALCOHOLIC BEVERAGES*

	corn	malt	rye	wheat	oats	rice	potato	grape	cactus	juniper	beet	cane	yeast
WHISKEY													
Bourbon	X	X	X	+	+	+		X			X	X	X
Blended bourbon	X	X	X	X	X	X	X	X			X	X	X
Canadian	X	X	X	X				X				X	X
Blended Canadian	X	X	X	X	X	X		X			X	X	X
Irish	X	X	X	X	X	X						X	X
Blended Irish	X	X	X	X	X	X		X			X	X	X
Scotch	X	X	+	+	+	+		X				X	X
Blended Scotch	X	X	X	X	X	X		X			X	X	X
GIN													
Grain spirits	X	X	X	+	+	+				X			X
Cane spirits	X	X	X	+	+	+				X		X	X
VODKA													
Domestic	X	X	X	X	+	+	+				+	+	X
Some imports							X						
RUM													
Domestic								X				X	X
Jamaican												X	X
TEQUILA	?								X				X
BEER	X	X	+	+	+	X					X	X	X
WINE													
Grape wine	+	+	+	+	+	+		X			+	+	X
Vermouth	+	+	+	+	+	+		X			+	+	X
Sherry	+	+	+	+	+	+		X			+	+	X
BRANDY	+							X			+	+	X
CORDIALS &													
LIQUEURS	X	X	X	X	+	+		X			X	X	X

* All commercially available liquors also contain various chemicals.

X Indicates most commonly employed source materials

+ Indicates permitted materials used sometimes

? Indicates material used rarely

SAMPLE ROTATION DIET (SRD)

This example of a ten day rotation diet is included to help
you put together an interesting diet while carefully rotating
foods.

Monday
Breakfast: arrowroot berry cobbler (p. 109)
            berry juice
Lunch: apple juice, cole slaw #2 (p. 74), apple slices
Dinner: grilled beef steak, barley casserole (p. 106)

Tuesday
Breakfast: hash-browned potatoes, orange slices, orange juice
Lunch: lettuce and avocado salad
Dinner: roasted chicken, steamed carrots (p. 67), three bean salad
            (p. 74)

Wednesday
Breakfast: baked squash with pineapple (p. 68), pineapple
            slices, pineapple juice
Lunch: cauliflower dipped in yogurt, cheese wedges
Dinner: grilled pork chop, wilted spinach (p. 67), pear
            sauce (p. 63)

Thursday
Breakfast: soy grits, figs
Lunch: tomato stuffed with egg salad (p. 73), celery sticks,
            tomato juice
Dinner: nut-fried fish (p. 75)

Friday
Breakfast: date-oat torte (p. 99)
Lunch: waldorf salad (p. 62), cashews, apple juice

Dinner: broiled lamb chop, steamed chard or broccoli
            (p. 67), mango slices

Saturday
Breakfast: buckwheat cereal (p. 108), stewed apricots (p. 63),
            apricot juice
Lunch: carrot salad (p. 73), grapefruit juice
Dinner: baked chicken, lettuce

Sunday
Breakfast: rice-berry cobbler (p. 92), berry juice
Lunch: squash casserole (p. 67-68), cheese wedges, chocolate
            ice cream (p. 89)
Dinner: sweet and sour pork (p. 82), pineapple slices, cole
            slaw #3 (p. 74)

Monday
Breakfast: soufflé (p. 84), nut squares (p. 86)
Lunch: oven-fried potatoes (p. 72), papaya wedges
Dinner: poached fish (p. 75), steamed asparagus (p. 67),
            celery sticks, watermelon ice (p. 65)

Tuesday
Breakfast: rye flakes (p. 95), figs
Lunch: lentil soup (p. 70), sliced mango
Dinner: grilled beef or lamb steak, steamed beets and greens
            (p. 67)

Wednesday
Breakfast: sweet potato pudding (p. 70-71), orange slices
Lunch: lettuce and avocado salad, persimmon slices
Dinner: chicken salad (p. 78), steamed carrots (p. 67),
            baked apple slices (p. 63)

BOTANICAL LIST OF FOOD FAMILIES

Foods, like people, come in families. Foods from the same family are so alike biologically that if you react to one food, you are likely to react to other foods in the same family.

Some of the relationships are startling. Did you know, for example, that tomatoes, peppers, tobacco and eggplant are all from the potato family? You may have noticed similarities between almonds and apricot seeds; they are close relatives. Garlic and asparagus are both found in the lily family. If you are allergic to poison ivy, you may also have difficulty with cashews.

If you are trying to control your allergic reactions by using a Rotation Diet, the following list is very important to you. In choosing your menu, be sure that you do not repeat a specific food more often than once every four days. Do not introduce another food from that same food family for at least 48 hours. To illustrate, apricots eaten on Monday may be followed by almonds on Wednesday.

Here are common members of food families:

Algae
  agar agar
  carrageen or Irish moss
  kelp or seaweed
Arrowroot (*Marantacae*)
  arrowroot (*Maranta* starch)
Arum (*Araceae*)
  ceriman (*Monstera*)
  dasheen (*Colocasia*)
  taro root (*Colocasia*) poi
  malanga (*Xanthosoma*)
  yautia (*Xanthosoma*)
Banana (*Fagaceae*)
  chestnut

Birch (*Betulaceae*)
  filbert
  hazelnut
  oil of birch or wintergreen

Borage (*Boraginaceae*)
  comfrey

Buckwheat (*Polygonaceae*)
  buckwheat
  garden sorrel
  rhubarb
  sea grape

Cactus (*Cactaneae*)
  prickly pear

Canna (*Cannaceae*)
Queensland arrowroot
Caper (*Capparidaceae*)
caper
Carpetweed (*Aizoaceae*)
New Zealand spinach
Carrot (*Umbelliferae*)
angelica
anise
caraway
carrot
chervil
celeriac, celery root
celery, celery seed
coriander
cumin
dill
fennel
finocchio
lovage
parsley
parsnip
sweet cicely
Cashew (*Anacardiaceae*)
cashew
mango
pistachio
poison ivy
poison oak
poison sumac
Composite (*Compositae*)
burdock root
camomile
cardoon
chicory root
dandelion
endive

escarole
globe artichoke
Jerusalem artichoke,
artichoke flour
kaffir
lettuce
safflower
santolina
southernwood
sunflower seed, oil
tansy
tarragon
wormwood or absinthe
yarrow
Conifer (*Coniferae*)
juniper
pine nut or piñon
Custard-apple (*Annonaceae*)
custard-apple (*Annona*
species)
papaw or pawpaw
Cycad (*Cycadaceae*)
Florida arrowroot (*Zamia*)
Ebony
kaki
persimmon
Flaxseed (*Linaceae*)
flaxseed
Fungi
baker's yeast
brewer's or nutritional yeast
mold (in certain cheeses),
citric acid (*Aspergillus*)
mushroom
puffball
truffle
Ginger (*Zingiberaceae*)

cardamon
East Indian arrowroot
ginger
turmeric
Goosefoot (*Chenopodiacae*)
  beet, beet sugar
  chard
  lamb's quarters
  spinach
  tampala
Gourd (*Cucurbitateae*)
  cantaloupe
  casaba melon
  chayote
  cucumber
  gherkin
  honeydew
  Persian melon
  pumpkin
  squash (acorn, butternut, caserta, cocozelle, crook-neck, hubbard, zucchini)
  watermelon
Grape (*Vitaceae*)
  grapes (brandy, champagne, cream of tartar, currants, raisins, wine, wine vinegar)
  muscadine
Grass (grain) (*Gramineae*)
  barley (malt, maltose)
  bamboo shoots
  corn (cornmeal, grits, hominy, corn oil, cornstarch, corn syrup)
  popcorn
  millet
  oat

rice
rye
sorghum
sugar cane (cane sugar, molasses, turbinado sugar)
wheat (bran, bulgur, gluten flour, graham flour, patent flour, semolina flour, whole wheat flour, wheat germ)
wild rice
Heath (*Ericaceae*)
  bearberry
  blueberry
  cranberry
  huckleberry
Holly (*Aquifoliacae*)
  mate
Honeysuckle (*Caprifoliaceae*)
  elderberry
Iris (*Iridaceae*)
  orris root
  saffron
Laurel (*Lauraceae*)
  avocado
  bay leaf
  cinnamon
  cassia
  sassafras
Legume (*Leguminosae*)
  alfalfa
  beans (fava, kidney, lima, mung and mung sprouts, navy, string)
  black-eyed pea (cowpea)
  carob
  chick-pea (garbanza)

fenugreek
lentil
licorice
pea
peanut (peanut oil)
soy (lecithin, soybean, soy
    flour, soy grits, soy milk,
    soy oil)
tonka bean (coumarin, vanilla
    flour)
Lily (*Liliaceae*)
  aloe vera
  asparagus
  chives
  garlic
  leek
  onion
  ramps
  shallot
  sarsaparilla
  yucca or soap plant
Linden (*Tiliaceae*)
  basswood, lime or linden
Madder (*Rubiaceae*)
  coffee
  woodruff
Mallow (*Malvaceae*)
  cotton seed meal, oil
  okra
Malpighia (*Malpighiaceae*)
  acerola or Barbados cherry
Maple (*Aceraceae*)
  maple sugar
  maple syrup
Mint (*Labiatae*)
  basil
  bergamot

catnip
clary
dittany
horehound
hyssop
lavender
lemon balm
marjoram
oregano
pennyroyal
peppermint
rosemary
spearmint
summer savory
thyme
winter savory
Mustard (*Cruciferae*)
  broccoli
  brussels sprouts
  cabbage
  cauliflower
  Chinese cabbage
  collards
  colza shoots
  horseradish
  kale
  kohlrabi
  mustard green
  mustard seed
  radish
  rape
  rutabaga or swede
  turnip
  upland cress
  watercress
Mulberry (*Moraceae*)
  breadfruit

fig
hop
mulberry
Myrtle (*Myrataceae*)
  allspice (*Pimenta*)
  clove
  eucalyptus
  guava
Nutmeg (*Myristicaceae*)
  mace
  nutmeg
Olive (*Oleaceae*)
  olive
Orchid (*Orchitaceae*)
  vanilla
Palm (*Palmaceae*)
  coconut (coconut meal, coconut oil)
  date (date sugar)
  palm cabbage
  sago starch (*Metroxylon*)
Papaya (*Caricaceae*)
  papaya
Passion-flower (*Passifloraceae*)
  granadilla or passion-fruit
Pedalium (*Pedaliaceae*)
  sesame seed (sesame seed flour, sesame seed oil)
Pepper (*Piperaceae*)
  black pepper
  peppercorn (*Piper*)
  white pepper
Pineapple (*Bromeliaceae*)
  pineapple
Pomegranate (*Puniceae*)
  grenadine
  pomegranate

Poppy (*Papaveraceae*)
  poppyseed
Potato (*Solanaceae*)
  eggplant
  ground cherry
  pepper (*Capsicum*)
    (cayenne, chili, paprika, pimento)
  potato
  tomato
  tobacco
Protea (*Proteaceae*)
  macadamia (Queensland nut)
Rose (*Roseaceae*)
pomes
  apple (cider, vinegar, pectin)
  pear
  quince
  rose hips
berries
  blackberry (boysenberry, dewberry, loganberry, youngberry)
  raspberry (black, red, purple)
  strawberry
  wineberry
stone fruits
  almond
  apricot
  nectarine
  peach
  plum (prune)
  sloe
Rue (*Citrus*)
  citron
  grapefruit
  kumquat

lemon
lime
orange
tangerine
tangelo
Sapodilla (*Sapotaceae*)
  chicle
Sapucaya nut (*Lecythidaceae*)
  Brazil nut
  sapucaya nut
Saxifrage (*Saxifragaceae*)
  currant
  gooseberry
Spurge (*Euphorbiaceae*)
  cassava or yucca
  tapioca or Brazilian arrowroot
Sterculia (*Sterculiaceae*)
  chocolate (cacao) (cocoa,
    cocoa butter)

cola (cola nut, coca-cola)

Tacca (*Traccaceae*)
  Fiji arrowroot (*Tacca*)

Tea (Theaceae)
  tea

Verbena (*Verbenaceae*)
  lemon verbena

Walnut (*Juglandaceae*)
  black walnut
  butternut
  English walnut
  heart nut
  hickory nut
  pecan

Yam (*Dioscoreaceae*)
  Chinese potato or yam

ANIMAL CLASSIFICATION AND MEAT FAMILIES

Amphibian
 frog
Crustacean (*Decapods*)
 crab
 crayfish
 lobster
 prawn
 shrimp
Fish: salt water
 anchovy
 bass (grouper)
 bluefish
 catfish
 codfish (cusk, haddock, pol-
  lack, scrod)
 croaker (drum, sea trout, silver
  perch, spot)
 dolphin
 eel
 flounder (dab, halibut, plaice,
  sole, turbot)
 mackerel (albacore, bonito,
  tuna)
 marlin (sailfish)
 mullet
 scorpionfish (ocean perch,
  rosefish)
 silverside
 swordfish
 tilefish
Fish: fresh water
 bass (white perch, yellow bass)

catfish
croaker (fresh-water drum)
herring (shad roe)
minnow (carp)
perch (sauger, walleye, yellow
 perch)
pike
salmon (trout)
sturgeon (caviar)
smelt
sucker (buffalo-fish)
sunfish (black bass, crappie)
whitefish
Mollusks
Gastropods
 abalone
 snail
Cephalopods
 squid
Pelecypods
 clam
 mussel
 oyster
 scallop
Fowl
 duck (goose)
 dove (pigeon, squab)
 grouse (partridge, ruffled
  grouse)
 pheasant (chicken, peafowl,
  pheasant, quail)
 guinea fowl

turkey
Mammals
  bear
  bovid
    beef cattle
      beef
      beef by-products (gelatin,
      oleomargarine, rennin or
      rennet, suet, sausage
      casings)
    milk products (butter, dried
    milk, ice cream, lactose,
    yogurt)
    veal
    buffalo or bison
    goat (cheese, milk)

sheep (lamb, mutton)
deer (caribou, elk, moose,
  reindeer)
hare (rabbit)
horse
opossum
pronghorn (antelope)
swine (hog or pork, bacon,
  ham, lard)
whale
gelatin
sausage
scrapple
Reptile
snake
turtle (terrapin)

RESOURCE READING LIST

Dickey, Lawrence D. *Clinical Ecology*. Springfield, Ill. Charles C. Thomas, 1976.

Frazer, Claude A. *Coping with Food Allergy*. New York: New York Times Book Company, 1974.

Golos, Natalie. *Management of Complex Allergies*. Norwalk, Conn. New England Foundation of Allergic and Environmental Diseases, 1975.

Hall, Kay Ludeman. "Allergy of the Nervous System: A Review." *Annals of Allergy*, vol. 36, pages 49–64, December 1975.

Hall, Ross Hume. *Food for Nought*. New York: Vintage Books, 1974.

Hills, Hilda Cherry. *Good Food, Gluten-Free*. New Canaan, CT.: Keats Publishing, Inc., 1976.

——— *Good Food, Milk-Free, Grain-Free*. New Canaan, CT.: Keats Publishing, Inc., 1979.

Mackarness, Richard. *Eating Dangerously*. New York and London: Harcourt Brace Jovanovich, 1976.

Miller, Joseph B. *Food Allergy Provocative Testing and Injection Therapy*. Springfield, Ill.: Charles C. Thomas, 1972.

O'Banion, Dan. *Academic Performance Affected by Sensitivities to Various Foods and Chemicals*. Center for Behavioral Studies, North Texas State University, Denton, Texas.

Pfeiffer, Carl C. *Mental and Elemental Nutrients*. New Canaan, CT.: Keats Publishing, Inc., 1975.

——— *Factbook on Zinc and Other Micronutrients*. New Canaan, CT.: Keats Publishing, Inc., 1978.

Randolph, T. G. *Human Ecology and Susceptibility to the Chemical Environment*. Springfield, Ill.: Charles C. Thomas, 1978.

Rea, William J. "Environmentally Triggered Small Vessel Vasculitis." *Annals of Allergy*, vol. 38, pages 245–257, April 19.

Selye, Hans. *The Stress of Life*. New York: McGraw-Hill Book Co. 1956.
Thie, John F., *Touch for Health*. Marina Del Rey, California: DeVorss and Co. 1973.

BIBLIOGRAPHY

Adcock, E.W., et al (1973). *Science* 181, 845–847.

Bardowil, W. A. and Toy, B.L. (1959). *Ann. of Acad. Sci.* 80 197–257.

Bellanti, J.A. (1971). *Immunology*. W.B. Saunders Co. Phil. PA., 69–90.

Braunstein, G.D., et al (1973), *Amer. J. Obstet. Gynec.* 115, 447–50.

Currie, G.A. and Bagshawe, K.D. (1967). *Lancet* 1, 708–710.

Jenkins, D.M., Acres, M.G., Petes, J. and Riley, J. (1972). *Am. J. Obstet. Gynec.* 114, 1315.

Jones, W.R. (1968). *Nature* 218, 480.

Kaye, M.D. and Jones, W.R. (1971). *Am. J. Obstet. Gynec.* 109, 1029–31.

Kirby, D.R.S., (1963). *J. Reprod. Fert.*, 5,1.

Kirby, D.R.S., (1967). *J. Reprod. Fert.*, 14, 515.

Kirby, D.R.S., (1968). *Adv. Reprod. Physio.* 3, 31.

Leikin, S. (1972). *Lancet* 2, 43.

Medawar, P.B. (1953). *Symp. Soc. Exp. Biol.*, vii, Evolution 320

Randolph, T.G. (1978). *Ann. Allergy*, 40, 5.

St. Hill, C.A., Finn, R. and Denye, V. (1973). *Brit. Med. J.* 3, 513–514.

Wynn, R.M. (1967). *Am. J. Obstet. Gynec.* 97, 832–850.

Index

Index

Louise Henderson, Ph.D., a psychologist and researcher, holds a Masters degree in clinical psychology and a doctorate in clinical behavioral medicine from the University of North Texas. She was introduced to the field of Human Ecology as a patient of Dr. Theron Randolph, a pioneer in environmentally triggered disease. She was a research assistant to William J. Rea, M.D., in Dallas for seven years. This close observation of the physical and psychological symptoms in food and chemical allergy patients led her to enter graduate studies in the field of psychology. Dr. Henderson completed her studies in 1984 and has been furthering her interests in the close interpersonal relationship of the family and research in the areas of breast cancer, Alzheimer's disease, multiple sclerosis and environmental illness. Her dissertation defining the environmentally ill patient for the professional was given special recognition in London in 1987 by the group Action Against Allergy. She was also recognized for community service by the Dallas Press Club in 1988. Dr. Henderson and her family recently moved to Evergreen, Colorado. Her next publication is in the area of the family and close interpersonal relationships as they pertain to illness.

Kate Ludeman, Ph.D., is a psychologist, corporate trainer, teacher, conference producer and researcher with a particular interest in nutrition. She holds degrees in psychology and engineering, and at present lectures on counseling and gerontology at Holy Name College, California. She has written several articles in professional journals, a section on "Orthomolecular Medicine and the Press" in Roger Williams's *Physician's Handbook on Orthomolecular Medicine* (reissued by Keats Publishing), and is working on a new book, *The Sexuality of the Older Woman*. She makes her home in San Francisco with her daughter Catherine.

Henry S. Basayne is a counselor, teacher and businessman. He is president of Educational Event Coordinators and a vice president of Manifest Learning Systems. He serves on the executive board of the Association for Humanist Psychology and chairs the Division of Humanist Counselors of the American Humanist Association. He lives in San Francisco.